Q.A.

QUALITY ASSURANCE IN LIBRARIES:

▲
THE
HEALTH
CARE
SECTOR
▼

A COLLECTION OF

STUDIES EDITED BY

MARGARET HAINES TAYLOR

AND TOM WILSON

Canadian Library Association
Library Association Publishing Limited

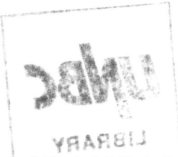

Canadian Cataloguing in Publication Data
Main entry under title:

Q.A. : quality assurance in libraries : the
    health care sector : a collection of studies

Co-published with: the Library Association.
ISBN 0-88802-255-7

    1. Quality assurance. 2. Medical libraries--
Evaluation. 3. Medical libraries--Standards.
I. Taylor, Margaret Haines. II. Wilson, Tom.
III. Canadian Library Association. IV. Library
Association. V. Title: Quality assurance in libraries.

Z678.85.Q28 1990   026'.61   C90-090539-5

British Library Cataloguing in Publication Data
Taylor, Margaret Haines
    Quality assurance in libraries : the health care sector
    1. Libraries. Performance. Assessment.
    I. Title   II. Wilson, Tom
    027

    ISBN 1-85604-006-2

Published by the Canadian Library Association
200 Elgin Street, Suite 602, Ottawa, Ontario K2P 1L5
Copyright © 1990 Canadian Library Association
All rights reserved
ISBN 0-88802-255-7

CONTENTS

DEDICATION

We dedicate this book to the memory of Mary Haines (1910-1990), who provided an inspiring example of optimism in the face of adversity.

Introduction

Quality

Quality is an elusive concept: we use the word a great deal in relation to all kinds of everyday things, but we find it difficult, often, to say exactly what it is about an object that gives it "quality". When we come to abstract ideas, such as "the quality of life" the problems are compounded — it becomes even more difficult to specify, in objective terms, what are the characteristics of a life of quality. Part of the difficulty lies in the fact that quality is a relative term. Advertisers use the word frequently to describe the products they promote: as a result, things of very different kinds may be said to be, for example, "quality cars", or "quality clothes". The concept of quality is related in these cases to another, rather vague idea, that of "value for money".

This book is about quality in a very particular context: the quality of library services, and here the same kind of problems exist as in trying to define quality in any other context. However, we can draw comparisons with other kinds of services: for example, the quality of service offered in shops and stores. When we go into a store we recognize quality in various ways: for example, the layout will be spacious and easy to move around; the signposting of different areas of the store will be unobtrusive but obvious and clear; the stock will be up-to-date and, in the food section, items past their sell-by date will have been removed; staff will be approachable and informative — they will know where goods of different kinds can be found and they will be able to advise the customer on appropriate products, guarantees offered, service availability and other matters; when an item is not available it can be ordered and will be delivered to one's home, or a telephone call will be made to let the customer know that it has arrived; and so on, and so on.

Clearly, each one of these characteristics of service quality in a store has a parallel in library services. A library, too, needs clean, spacious, and well-organized areas for use by clients; it needs effective signposting of the different areas of stock; the stock itself should be up-to-date and regularly weeded of items past their useful life; staff should be approachable (in the jargon of the day, they should have good interpersonal skills) and knowledgeable about the stock and the range of services offered; effective and responsive reservation and inter-library loan services should exist; and where the library serves a closed population, it should be possible for a client to have an item delivered to his or her desk. In these days of online, public-access catalogues it should also be possible for such clients to consult the catalogue at their desks.

These attributes of the *quality library* have been known for almost as long as the open-access library has existed, if not longer, and yet we are still, apparently, in the situation of needing to reinforce these ideas. We can all point to services that exhibit shortcomings in respect of the quality characteristics just described and, in the UK, in the public sector, many libraries are finding it very difficult to maintain quality because of the lack of financial resources. Ironically, the shortage of money is the result of a government determination to get better "value for money" out of the expenditure on public services.

Quality assurance

There is a need, therefore, for librarians to take positive steps to assure the client of the quality of the services offered. And it is well to think of what the word *assure* means: it means that a guarantee is being offered, a promise that the library services will meet client needs, as expeditiously as possible, and in physical surroundings that will make library use as pleasing an experience as shopping in the best department store in town.

The ultimate aim, therefore, of a quality assurance plan, is to make it possible for the librarian to assure clients that the services offered are of a good quality, *within the limits of the budget.* This is an important caveat to enter because in many situations the library's clients may have a role in determining the library budget. If they want higher quality than can be afforded within the present budget, they must be informed of the fact, so that the librarian can influence future decision-making in which the clients play a part.

The measurement problem

Given the nature of the characteristics of quality, it is not surprising that they are difficult to measure. This does not mean that they are difficult to recognize or to *assess*. It is a relatively easy matter to look at two stores and to come away with a subjective impression of their relative quality: we can do the same with two libraries, simply through walking into them and looking around, and, in more depth, by making comparative use of them. The whole area of non-obtrusive testing of reference services, for example, shows that quality testing is possible.

However, there is certainly a difficulty in finding objective, numeric measures for some of the characteristics of quality. Or, if not in finding the measures, then in affording the time necessary to collect the relevant data. If we look back at the characteristics listed earlier it will be evident that some matters *can* be judged in objective terms, while others are amenable only to subjective assessment. For example: it is possible to measure the response time of a request for an inter-library loan or a reservation, and Richard Orr and his colleagues at the Institute for the Advancement of Medical Communication developed the *document delivery test* as a means of measuring the ability of a library to deliver the documents likely to be needed by clients a good many years ago. We can also assess how useful the stock of a library is by collecting data on which items are borrowed, or used in the library, and which items remain unused on the shelf. Enough data now exists on use patterns to enable us to make management decisions on the removal of items from the shelf, either to a reserve stack or out of the library altogether. With modern, computer-based, library management systems it ought to be possible to turn the task of weeding into a relatively mechanical process by flagging all items in the catalogue that have not been used for a particular period of time.

Clearly, however, some characteristics of quality cannot be "measured" in this way. For example, the quality of staff must be assessed by more subjective methods. In large part this is a matter of effective internal training programmes and effective supervision. Unobtrusive testing can be used, but there is a certain ethical problem caused by the distasteful idea of "spying" upon one's work colleagues. However, surveys of client satisfaction, particularly if these are done by interviewing clients in their own settings, rather than in the library, can provide a great deal of instructive, critical comment.

Performance measurement

There is, of course, an entire literature devoted to one aspect of quality assurance, that is, performance measurement. However, the distinction must be drawn between performance measurement and quality assurance: quality assurance is an attempt to guarantee the quality of service offered by a library or information service — the aim is to decide, in advance, what quality of service one can afford, and then to seek to achieve that degree of quality. In other words, quality assurance is an attempt to define how well you want to perform. Performance measurement, on the other hand, attempts to measure how well you have done. On its own, performance measurement is no guarantee of anything: it only serves a really useful, managerial purpose when it is allied to the kind of objectives setting activity that is an essential part of quality assurance.

All too often, in seeking measures of performance, library managers fall back upon the tried and trusted means of data collection from the records they keep of their activities. Thus, loan records are used, because they are simple to collect; or records of the books added to stock are allied to figures of potential or actual user population, giving ratios that indicate at least some kind of recognition of user needs. *Real* performance measures, however, will attempt to measure outcomes of service, rather than inputs or processes, but it is much more difficult to do this than it is to collect data on transactions and processes.

Of course, some ratios will be indicative of the level of service offered. There is a kind of basic common-sense about ratios such as the number of journals per user, or the number of inter-library loans acquired per user: these measures do relate to an attempt on the part of the library to satisfy user needs. More imagination, however, and a greater acceptance of the fact that numbers can be manipulated to provide support for almost anything, is needed if librarians are to begin to identify the outcome measures that will persuade senior managers of the validity of their cases for more resources.

The quality manager

This last point illustrates one of the essential desiderata of the quality library: a quality manager. Ultimately, the quality of library service depends upon the imagination, commitment and managerial qualities of the librarian. Only the library manager can motivate others to deliver quality service, can insist upon quality performance by his/her subordinates, can operate effectively within the organization to win the resources necessary to ensure that a quality job can be done. To operate effectively as a manager demands the acquisition of managerial skills against those of the professional librarian and simply because one has been good at the tasks demanded of the latter is no guarantee that a person can perform effectively in a managerial role. A library manager must have sufficient self-analytical ability to know when s/he needs further training in one or other of the many skills demanded of today's professional manager.

Quality Assurance in Health Sector Libraries

Quality managers are as important in health libraries as they are in any other organization or library. In some respects, health librarians are fortunate that they work in a public service culture which has already embraced the concepts of quality assurance, quality improvement, total quality management, etc. Thus, their efforts to develop quality library services must be in harmony with quality improvement efforts elsewhere in the health sector.

The concern for quality in health care facilities originated in the North American hospital accreditation movement of the early 1900's when the American College of Surgeons launched a movement to set standards by which a hospital's efficiency could be measured (Greeniaus, 1985). Following the work of the ACS in measuring hospital performance, several organizations such as the Joint Commission on the Accreditation of Hospitals in the U.S.A. and the Canadian Council for Hospital Accreditation were formed to promote and encourage an optimal quality of health care by the achievement of accreditation standards in all hospitals and related health care organizations.

Standards for libraries have been included in the North American accreditation standards since the 1950's and have focussed on collection development, space and facilities, budgets, interlibrary loans, and even occasionally on library staff. While the scope and detail of these library standards have varied considerably over the years, they have improved with time through increased communication between the accreditation bodies and the professional health library associations.

The accreditation standards did not address the issue of "evaluating" whether quality was being achieved until the late 1970s and early 1980s when they emphasized that a health care facility's quality assurance programme would affect the accreditation of that facility. The term "quality assurance" was generally agreed to mean the establishment of hospital-wide goals, the assessment of procedures to determine whether these goals are being achieved and, if not, the proposal of means to attain these goals. For many librarians, this was the beginning of their involvement with QA. Indeed, in Canada, the standards for libraries included a requirement that "there shall be procedures established to evaluate the quality of library services and performance of personnel" (Canadian Council of Hospital Accreditation, 1983).

The task then faced by most health librarians in North America is one which is facing many of their colleagues in the UK now: how to cope with this concept of "quality assurance": how to relate quality assurance for the library to organization wide programmes and vice versa; how to conduct "QA" activities when understaffed and overworked already; how far to equate quantitative criteria with quality of service; how to cope with the absence of meaningful and concise criteria for library functions; how to decide where to begin and what to evaluate; and how to cope with a lack of consensus in what "quality" and "QA" in the library means. (Duchow, 1985).

This task is not an easy one but obtaining information from librarians engaged in the process, whether on a one-to-one basis, through the literature or at professional meetings, does seem to help. Most librarians who have been through the "QA" process agree that it is hard work, frustrating, challenging, edifying and satisfying. It is often the first real test of their management skills as opposed to their professional skills and as a result of their efforts implementing "QA", they improve their own abilities for setting goals and objectives, for weighing priorities, for creative and lateral thinking in problem solving and for lobbying for increased resources.

The impact of quality assurance on health librarianship has been felt in a number of other key areas: increased networking between librarians, improved standards and accreditation tools, increased awareness of librarianship within the health care management community, and most important, improved library services. With this in mind, every librarian should feel encouraged to try to develop a quality assurance programme. This book has been developed to help share the knowledge gained by other librarians who have tried to assure quality in their library services.

The Plan of This Book

We begin the book with a chapter on strategic planning which is the first step in developing missions, goals and objectives upon which QA programmes can be based. The next two chapters describe professional association activities in Canada and Europe relating to the development of standards for health libraries which can be used in QA programmes. Goals, objectives and standards are not the only ingredients for a successful QA programme and thus the next two chapters focus on the need for appropriate data collection methods and the problem of performance measures. Following this, three chapters discuss how QA has been used in a variety of essential library functions: reference services, interlibrary loans, and collection development. The final chapters describe QA programmes in the specialized settings of a consumer health information service, and a quality assurance information service.

Acknowledgements

As editors we are glad to acknowledge the contributions of our colleagues in providing the individual papers. All of the authors are busy people, all trying to provide quality services, often under difficult and trying circumstances. Without them the collection could not have existed. We would also like to thank colleagues, family and friends on both sides of the Atlantic who constantly encouraged us to see this work through. We also acknowledge the patience of our publisher who must have wondered at times whether the promised camera-ready copy was ever going to materialize. Finally, we must acknowledge the relatively trouble-free hardware and software that produced the camera-ready copy: a Viglen SL3 386SX microcomputer, an HP Laserjet III printer, and the software packages WordPerfect and LaTeX.

MHT & TDW

References

Canadian Council for Hospital Accreditation. (1983) *Standards for Accreditation of Canadian Health Care Facilities.* Ottawa, CCHA.

Duchow, S. (1985) Quality assurance for health and hospital libraries: general considerations and background. *Bibliotheca Medica Canadiana,* **6,** 177–181.

Greeniaus, B. (1985) The Canadian Council on Hospital Accreditation: a brief history. *Bibliotheca Medica Canadiana,* **6,** 130–135.

Strategic planning: the basis for quality assurance

Dorothy Fitzgerald
Librarian, Health Sciences Library, McMaster University, Hamilton, Ontario, Canada.

Introduction

To be fully effective, quality assurance must be undertaken in the context of a total programme of improvement in the delivery of library services through planning and implementation, training, public relations, and performance monitoring. This paper presents a case study in the first stage of such a programme: strategic planning. The focus of the study is an academic health sciences library. Developing and implementing strategy offer tremendous opportunities for organizational learning and it is with this in mind that the McMaster experience is provided. The case focuses on the process and model used by this library, to illustrate both the benefits experienced and the lessons learned. As part of this study, the organizational structure and environment of the McMaster University Health Sciences Library are described. The study ends with an outline of current activities and the necessary next stage in this evolving planning process, as seen from the Library's perspective.

In these times of tremendous and rapid change in the information world, together with fiscal constraints placed on universities and hospitals, libraries are working to improve their ability to cope with uncertainty and change and learning a great deal in the process. Of particular interest to health sciences librarians is the new discipline of medical informatics which, broadly defined, combines medical science with technologies and disciplines in the information and computer sciences to provide methodologies for the management of information to support medical research, education, and patient care (Matheson, 1990). The landmark study by Matheson and Cooper considers potential roles for the library in information management (Matheson 1982). The GPEP Report, aimed at reorienting the emphasis in medical education, recommends that medical schools "designate an academic unit for institutional leadership in the application of information sciences and computer technology to the general professional education of physicians and promote their effective use." (GPEP Report, 1984) The role of the library in the educational process, in terms of promoting information literacy (the ability to find, evaluate and use information effectively) is receiving attention on a broad scale (Breivik and Gee, 1989). Strategic planning, an approach adopted by many libraries to deal with these exciting and challenging developments, has been simply defined as an attempt to look ahead to where you want to be, coupled with a program to get you there (Sheldon, 1989).

In terms of the purpose of the planning exercise undertaken at McMaster, Andrews provides a very useful view of corporate strategy as:

> "the pattern of major objectives, purposes, or goals and essential policies and plans for achieving those goals, stated in such a way as to define what business the company is in or is to be in and the kind of company it is or is to be. In a changing world it is a way of expressing a persistent concept of the business so as to exclude some possible new activities and suggest entry into others." (Andrews, 1971)

McMaster University. Faculty of Health Sciences

The central tenets of the Faculty, articulated as a result of its 1988-89 strategic planning process begin:

> "We are a Faculty of Health Sciences characterized by interdisciplinary, interprofessional, interfaculty and inter-institutional cooperation, working to achieve our goals of excellence in education, research and service." (*Tenets...*, 1990)

Programmes are based on a definition of health which incorporates biological, psychological and social well-being and focuses not only on the treatment of disease but on the promotion of health and the prevention of illness.

While the programmes in the Faculty use a variety of teaching/learning approaches, emphasis is placed on small group, problem-based learning with a focus on acquisition of critical appraisal skills. The Faculty values a community approach to health care, characterized by participation, responsiveness and responsibility shared with partner agencies and institutions.

The Faculty offers undergraduate degree programmes in medicine, nursing, occupational therapy and physiotherapy, postgraduate (Internship and Residency) education programmes; M.Sc., Ph.D. and post-professional programmes in a number of areas.

The Health Sciences Centre at McMaster University, which officially opened in 1972, houses both the Faculty of Health Sciences and a 300 bed teaching hospital (the McMaster Division of Chedoke-McMaster Hospitals). Many Faculty activities are established in cooperation with community hospitals and other health agencies. Satellite programmes at institutions in Northwestern Ontario continue to expand.

The Health Sciences Library, located in the Health Sciences Centre, occupies 40,000 sq. ft. on two levels and is one of three main libraries on the McMaster University campus. The Director of this Library reports to the Vice-President, Health Sciences and maintains a line of communication with the University Librarian. There are nine librarians and 24 full-time equivalent support staff. While the Director meets with the Head of Systems and Technical Services and the Head of Public Services frequently as the executive committee, the Library's Management Committee meets every two weeks to share information and discuss general policy issues. This committee is composed of all librarians on staff and the two professional management positions. In addition to the full range of public and technical services, the Library administers a Health Library Network programme with a membership of six hospital libraries and eight health agency libraries. Based on a funding formula, the Library serves as the hospital library for the McMaster Division of the Chedoke-McMaster Hospitals. This twenty year old Library continues to have an open and attractive atmosphere even though it is now facing serious space problems. The Library subscribes to 1,825 current journals and adds approximately 3,600 books, audio-visual and software programmes to the collection each year.

As the major learning resource for educational programmes with a philosophy of problem-based, self-directed learning, the Library is heavily used by the students. The 600 seats are often fully occupied as the Library has one of the highest gate counts for North American medical libraries (close to 600,000 in 1989-90). Circulation figures reflect the heavy use of the collection with over 122,000 reserve loans and 50,000 regular loans in 1989/90.

Students in this educational environment are strongly encouraged to use the journal literature and the five CD-ROM workstations in the Library are extremely popular. A priority project for 1990/91 is implementation of remote and multi-user access to Medline on CD-ROM. Direct searching using Greatful Med software is extremely popular in Hamilton as a result of the McMaster studies on end-user searching (Haynes, 1990). However, students continue to prefer online searching where no costs are incurred. A 15% drop in the number of search requests done by librarians has been experienced each year for the past three years; however, formal and informal instruction and assistance with end-user searching has increased substantially.

The Educational Microcomputer Laboratory, in the multi-media resource area of the Library, provides ten microcomputers connected to the University's Ethernet network, and a collection of computer assisted instruction packages. Overall, the Library has increased its complement of microcomputers from three in 1984 to forty in 1990 with fifteen available for public use and twenty-five available for staff use. Campus wide implementation of the integrated library system NOTIS, to be available to users in September 1990, will increase this number substantially. Most microcomputers are connected to the ethernet network which links computers throughout the Faculty and the University, and provides access to Netnorth. Vaxmail is used to facilitate communication both within the Library and externally.

In 1987 the Health Sciences Library embarked on a strategic planning process which continues to evolve today. This approach to planning was adopted in response to the extremely fast pace of change which was being experienced by Library staff. It was decided that a formal mechanism was needed to focus the efforts of the Library to meet the changing and expanding needs of its user community. It was accepted that an organization must evolve toward an appropriate planning approach and that it must involve the staff who make the Library work on a day-to-day basis. There are many models in the literature which describe the strategic planning activities of large and complex organizations (King, 1981). While many of the basic concepts and premises are generally applicable, it is possible and perhaps more appropriate to use a simple and straightforward model for a relatively small organization, such as this Health Sciences Library.

The Planning Process : Phase 1

By February 1987 the pace of change and the number of new challenges and opportunities being experienced by the Librarians suggested the need for a better mechanism to decide on Library priorities. The Director decided to formalize the process from the beginning by conveying the importance that would be placed on this initiative by management, and the expectation that this would be a major time-consuming organizational activity. It was recognized that the first step would be involvement of the members of the Library's Management Committee. Drawing on experience with strategic planning, both as a board member of the Canadian Health Libraries Association (CHLA) and as a tutor in the organization studies course offered in the Faculty, the Director chose a strategic planning model which requires that an organization define its mission, goals and objectives as a means of providing direction. Background readings and CHLA examples were provided to clarify the use of strategic planning terminology for our purposes. (Charns, 1983) In preparation for the initial strategic planning meeting members were asked to briefly document their view of what the Library's ten most important goals should be. This material was consolidated and circulated before the first meeting. The intent of that meeting was to brainstorm, using the suggested goals as a focus. During the meeting it became obvious that there would be many *process* issues to deal with, given the variety of personalities and levels of expertise available in this group of ten people. Immediate recognition and open discussion of the potential for difficult group dynamics in this process proved to be helpful in the long-term.

The many suggested goals fit easily into six broad topics: access, education, cooperation, innovation, staff and collections. Some suggested goals were really environmental factors affecting the Library; financial constraints and new technology were two examples of this kind. With some members thinking in much more specific terms than others, the difficulty in consistent use of the terms goals and objectives had begun. The mission statement of the Library as it had appeared in annual reports for a number of years was examined and found to be lacking. Refinement of that statement would also require careful consideration.

During the next couple of months members of the Management Committee worked in groups of three to develop goal statements for the six topics identified in the first meeting. *Goals* were seen as specific statements of results: targets toward which effort and action can be directed. In true Faculty of Health Sciences fashion, small groups met to brainstorm and then bring ideas back to the large group in order to reach broad consensus. The resulting goals statements (Tables 1 and 2) provided a framework for the next stage in formulating a strategy.

In June 1987, four months after the process had begun, the Committee again broke up into groups of three to meet as often as necessary to work on objectives. It was decided that all three small groups would work on *access* objectives as a trial run, to ensure that all members were on the same wavelength in terms of the meaning of the word objective in the context of this planning process. This proved to be a difficult stage as objectives generated in these small groups ranged from extremely broad to very narrow statements. At this point some members were ready to throw in the towel and stop trying to use terms such as goals and objectives consistently. Not everyone had taken ownership of the process and some convincing was required to maintain the momentum. One of the senior Librarians had recently attended a Medical Library Association continuing education course on Strategic Planning. She noted that while use of the terms mission, goals and objectives in the course was compatible with the Library's use, the course had suggested another possible layer of statements, specific *action plans*, below objectives. The model she presented incorporated many of the ideas generated about environmental factors and allowed for documentation of very specific activities. As a result, it made sense to the group in the context of the work they had been doing. Definitions provided by this model are:

- **Mission:** broad statement of purpose justifying the library's existence.

- **Goals:** qualitative statements which collectively describe the conditions existing when the library is fulfilling its mission.

- **Objectives:** specific results or ends, which are essential to fulfillment of the library's goals.

- **Action Plans:** specific activities, for which the responsibilities and resources can be assigned and a mutually agreed upon target date can be established. The sum of these activities equals the results necessary for attainment of specific objectives. (Braude 1983)

June and July of 1987 saw a great deal of activity on the part of the small groups in grappling with access objectives. One side benefit to this

Health Sciences Library McMaster University

MISSION STATEMENT

The primary mandate of the library is to support the educational, research and clinical programs conducted by and for the faculty, students and staff of the McMaster University Faculty of Health Sciences. The library is also a resource for the McMaster Division of the Chedoke McMaster Hospitals; other McMaster University faculties; the Hamilton-Wentworth Health Library Network; the Northwestern Ontario Medical Programme and the McMaster Health Region.

ACCESS GOAL: To provide efficient and effective access through tools and services which interpret and make available health sciences and related information from library collections and other sources.

COLLECTIONS GOAL: To provide and maintain a quality collection which supports and anticipates the educational, research and clinical needs of the community of users served by the Library.

COOPERATION GOAL: To promote cooperative attitudes and to establish and maintain cooperative relationships which foster the mission of the Library.

EDUCATION GOAL: To provide learning opportunities and resources which assist users in developing efficient and effective skills in accessing and organizing information.

INNOVATION GOAL: To apply and/or develop new methods of organizational management and information handling and retrieval in order to deliver improved services to users and staff.

STAFF GOAL: To provide a qualified and motivated staff in sufficient numbers to carry out Library services and activities.

Table 1: Mission and goals

ACCESS GOAL:

TO PROVIDE EFFICIENT AND EFFECTIVE ACCESS THROUGH
TOOLS AND SERVICES WHICH INTERPRET AND MAKE
AVAILABLE HEALTH SCIENCES AND RELATED INFOR-
MATION FROM LIBRARY COLLECTIONS AND OTHER SOUR-
CES.

OBJECTIVES:

1. To produce a record for every item held by the Library.

2. To produce a catalogue which includes records for all types of material
   held by the Library.

3. To acquire tools which offer access to worldwide health related information, such as indexes and abstracts, bibliographies, catalogues and
   databases.

4. To produce quality access tools which supplement the acquired tools.

5. To provide interlibrary loan and other services to obtain material not
   held by the Library.

6. To provide quality reference and orientation services to assist and train
   users in accessing information, in order to maximize their independence.

7. To provide reasonable hours of opening and emergency access when
   closed, reprographic services, appropriate space and equipment and
   stack maintenance.

8. To provide circulation and reserve services with loan periods and policies which give users equal access to library resources.

9. To evaluate periodically all services and tools which provide access.

Table 2: Access goal and objectives

exercise, not to be underestimated, was the necessity of the members of the Management Committee to take time the better to understand the concerns and priorities of staff in all areas of the Library. Reference staff had to grapple with the kinds of problems faced by the head of cataloguing and vice versa. A Management Committee composed of many strong-willed, extremely competent and determined people at times tested the mettle of some members.

For the more junior Librarians and the professional management staff on the committee, it was a revelation that there could be such strong feeling about the very nature of the Library catalogue. Well intentioned objectives such as "to provide universal access to all materials in the Library" provoked heated discussion. Unfortunately such issues were not always easily resolved as at times extreme positions were taken and little listening occurred. This is the reality of taking a close look at the details of an organization and needs to be accepted as such. Every effort was made to help group members see alternate points of view and express opposition in a way that was not threatening to the person making the suggestion. This human dynamics component of the strategic planning process was extremely valuable to the Library in general terms, as improved mechanisms for open debate have resulted and benefit the overall operation of the Library. Management Committee members gained a much clearer understanding of the multitude of issues facing staff in areas of the Library where they do not normally spend their time.

In many ways selecting the Access Goal as the test run in terms of having all members struggle with developing objectives was the right decision as this goal encompasses the functions of most areas of the Library. As indicated in Table 2, issues related to the catalogue, interlibrary loans, seating, circulation, reference, and online services are covered in this goal. It is true that tempers flared and frustration was evident, but it is also true that members were by now seriously committed to the process and saw the value in carrying on.

During the next four months Management Committee members again arranged to meet as necessary in predetermined groups of three to work on objectives for the other five goals. The education and innovation goals generated interesting discussion and again served as an educational experience for members of the Management Committee. In fact it was the new educational roles that the Librarians were taking on that had in part precipitated this process in the first place. A number of the Librarians were working with groups in the Faculty to teach not only traditional bibliographic skills but

also skills related to the general use of microcomputers for electronic communication and use in personal filing systems. The information management
and computer expertise of the Librarians were recognized by colleagues in
the Faculty with resulting invitations to be involved in Faculty-wide initiatives to introduce students and Faculty to computers. In terms of the
innovation goal, Librarians were taking leading roles in the Faculty to assist
in the planning for an Ethernet network. They played a significant role in
introducing an electronic conferencing system to the campus.

But what priority do these initiatives have in relation to the day-to-day
issues of running the Library? This was a valuable time for open discussion
on these sensitive issues. An important influence when considering the innovation goal was the culture of the Faculty of Health Sciences. This Faculty
prides itself on taking an innovative approach to endeavours, particularly
in relation to its educational programmes. The Health Sciences Library is
very much an integral part of the Faculty and it was always intended that
the strategic plan of the Library would be compatible with the goals of the
Faculty. When the Faculty began its strategic planning in 1988 the Library
was able to ensure that the goals of both were compatible. The Faculty
is very involved in international activities and Librarians have been invited
to participate in certain projects to provide both telecommunications and
information management expertise to medical schools in developing countries. These are clearly interesting and valuable initiatives, but, again, when
and under what circumstances do they tie in with the overall goals of the
Library? These were all important issues that needed to be addressed and
the strategic planning process was providing a useful mechanism for the discussions to take place. These issues also provide examples of the Library's
attempt continually to scan the environment to ensure that its strategy was
being developed in relation to internal and external environmental forces.

After nine months of strategic planning by the Management Committee
it was decided that it was time to solicit input from all Library staff and the
Health Sciences Library Users Committee.

While the various groups were reviewing the Draft Mission, Goals and
Objectives document, the Management Committee moved on to the next
stage in the process: development of action plans. These statements were
to reflect very specific actions to be completed by a certain date. To get
the ball rolling the full committee worked on the action plans for the access

objectives. While this exercise proved to be useful and straightforward this was not the case when the members once again broke up into small groups to develop action plans for the other goals. Widespread group discussion was required on how realistic some action plans were and who should be responsible to see that they happen. In a sense, there was an element of peer review occurring when, for example, individuals who were expected to take responsibility for certain projects were reluctant to do so.

Discussion was required to uncover why the project was seen as a priority for some Management Committee members and not by the person responsible for that function in the Library. While it was not always a comfortable situation, departmental managers had to accept the positive and negative aspects of participative management. At this stage in the process it was agreed that the document would include only those activities that were not already taking place in the Library. Activities which were considered important but were already a regular part of Library operations were excluded. This had to be explained clearly to people not involved in developing the document; otherwise feedback could focus on ongoing activities which had been excluded. It became increasingly clear however that this approach was causing difficulty as no parallel review of ongoing functions was taking place.

A full-day retreat for the entire library staff was scheduled for June 1988 to provide an open forum for review and discussion of the plan. This event provided the impetus to finalizing the document for circulation to staff prior to June. The retreat proved to be extremely valuable to the staff. It took place a year and a half after the planning process had begun. By this time the members of the Management Committee were very committed to the planning process and could comfortably confirm in their presentations at the retreat that it was a valuable exercise. Part of the day was devoted to small group discussions of two issues contained in the plan. The staff development issue generated forty-two suggestions or questions for consideration by the Management Committee. The second issue dealt with concerns about the Educational Microcomputer Laboratory and these small group discussions generated forty-three questions and suggestions and resulted in a Task Force being established to address them.

In many ways the retreat can be seen as the completion of phase one of the strategic planning process. The retreat was a very successful finale for the members of the Management Committee who had been working on the strategic plan for sixteen months by this time. The summer of 1988 was understandably a quiet time in terms of follow-up to the retreat and gearing up for phase two.

The Planning Process: Phase 2

The Fall of 1988, the second year in the process, was a time to review action plans with a view to ensuring that target dates were met. In some ways the plan and the meetings to review progress served as a tickler file to remind people that they had committed themselves to focusing on certain priorities. The Director set the pace for the frequency of meetings and, thereby, indicated the level of importance that was being given to the process.

Strategic planning will never allow a Library to anticipate every threat and opportunity. It became clear, as meetings to review action plans continued, that new developments were having a major impact on the Library and had to be tied into the strategic planning discussions which tended to focus on the document as finalized in May 1988.

Early in 1989, the third year in the process, a date was set for the second annual retreat. Setting the date again gave committee members a renewed impetus to remain on top of their action plans, as a primary purpose of the retreat was to report to staff on the progress that had been made on action plans with target dates to June 1989, the date of the retreat. In reality, discussions at the retreat also dealt with the current environment, developments which could not have been anticipated when the "plan" was being developed.

The Cycle begins again

In early 1990 the Management Committee, with four new members who had not participated in the development of the plan, decided that the first step in the renewal phase was to take a fresh look at the mission statement and the goals and objectives and determine if in fact they were still relevant.

It was agreed that the strategic planning process, as carried out to 1989, had been extremely worthwhile, both in formulating clearly articulated goals and objectives for the Library, and in improving the ability of the Management Committee to work as a team. However, this planning process had not been linked closely enough to the decision-making process to maximize our ability to make an impact on the Library's organizational effectiveness. Certainly, new opportunities or challenges were reviewed with the strategic plan as a guide. For example, the Librarians agreeing to taking on major roles in planning the 1991 annual conference of the Canadian Health Libraries Association was considered in this manner. However, the problem is that the strategic plan as a free standing document with specific action plans is necessarily out of date as soon as it is printed and it is virtually impossible to keep such a detailed plan up to date in any meaningful way. The document, when used as a *guide* however, is a useful mechanism for reviewing new projects and accepting or rejecting them based on their value in terms of the Library's goals and objectives.

The mission, goals and objectives document was seen by the Management Committee as an extremely valuable statement. It was seen that it could be used to make further impact on organizational effectiveness by affecting decision-making related to the ongoing services and operations in the Library. The increasing demand for services and resources, the new opportunities presented by information technology, and the impact of our improved acquisitions budget were demanding improved methods of making decisions about the allocation of scarce resources.

It was seen that more information was needed to link our ongoing planning process to the decision-making process in a way that would maximize the effectiveness of the Library. McClure's action research model addresses this need and recognizes the importance of integrating research with planning and decision-making (Swisher and McClure, 1984). In fact, McClure suggests that a goal in and of itself might be: to obtain knowledge that can be directly applied to the Health Sciences Library to increase organizational effectiveness.

As a result of our strategic planning activity our management team now recognizes that research is necessary to acquire the necessary information to affect planning and decision making. Traditional assumptions about services and resources must now be tested against the accepted goals and objectives of the Library. Since all services and operations cannot realistically be subjected to analysis and review, given the pressures of running the Library, mechanisms must be found to select for review those operations which have the greatest impact on the effectiveness of the Library. Problems selected for study must be directly linked to the goals and objectives of the Library, and decisions related to reviewing the problem must have the potential to have a major impact on the effectiveness of the Library. An example of a potential area for study would be the issue of staffing the Reference Desk with professional librarians. Is this model of staffing the desk the most effective use of staff resources in terms of the overall effectiveness of the Library? Involvement in this research activity will require that Library projects be reviewed, and certain projects be put on the back burner so that this activity can become a priority. A stage beyond studying the value of selected Library services and operations is to review how well they are done. Performance measures will be useful in this aspect of analysis.

In retrospect we consider that the time and energy invested in the strategic planning process was very worthwhile. It is extremely helpful for a library to have a clearly stated mission, goals and objectives document which includes a preamble to outline the organizational, political and economic environment of the Library. Developing this document as we did, with the total involvement of a major segment of the staff, was beneficial from all perspectives. This group of 10, our Management Committee, is, as a result, totally committed to the document and sees it as a useful guide to decision making.

What would we do differently? Basically the work to formulate our mission, goals and objectives was done in the first year of the process. We then decided to continue on to develop "action plans" using this same Management Committee as the forum. This proved to be extremely time consuming and difficult to keep up to date. Given the rapid rate of change in libraries today, it is really impossible to keep an accurate and up to date list of specific activities. This level of decision-making is better handled at the departmental level, with broad general policy issues brought to the Management Committee for information, and for discussion and consensus when appropriate. The mission, goals and objectives document can serve as a guide to all departments in developing their action plans. Perhaps the Library's Annual Report is more realistically the place to record success in meeting departmental action plans.

During our planning process we focused on new initiatives when considering action plans. Ongoing activities were not subject to review. Given fiscal constraints this is no longer possible. We now recognize the need to evaluate existing programmes and services to ensure that we are using our scarce resources to the maximum benefit. Time and effort might have been better spent on this evaluation work than the extensive group work of formulating action plans. A first step has been taken in this evaluation process. Meetings with key individuals (library departmental representatives and departmental chairmen) are being used to obtain information needed to update our Collections Policy and to get general feedback on library services and resources. A one page questionnaire listing the library's 17 key services and resources is being used to obtain feedback on the perceived importance and quality of these 17 areas. Following an analysis of feedback from this select group the questionnaire, fine tuned if necessary, will be used to obtain feedback from a much wider segment of our user population. In parallel with this activity selected services will be evaluated in depth from the perspective of both effectiveness and efficiency. This improved linking of our planning process with our decision making process should enhance organizational effectiveness and continue to encourage organizational learning.

References

Andrews, K.R. (1971) *The concept of corporate strategy.* Homewood, Ill.: Irwin.

Braude, R.M. (1983) *CE 258: Planning – strategic and tactical.* Chicago, Ill.: Medical Library Association.

Breivik, P.S. and Gee, E.G. (1989) *Information literacy: revolution in the library.* New York N.Y.: Macmillan.

Charns, M.P. and Schaefer, M.J. (1983) *Health care organizations: a model for management.* Englewood Cliffs N.J.: Prentice-Hall.

GPEP Report. (1984) *Physicians for the Twenty-First Century: report of the Panel on the General Professional Education of the Physician and College Preparation for Medicine.* Washington, D. C.: Association of American Medical Colleges.

Haynes, R.B., et al. (1990) Online access to MEDLINE in clinical settings: a study of use and usefulness. *Annals of Internal Medicine,* **112,** 78-84.

King, W.R. (1981) Strategic planning for public service institutions. What can be learned from business? *Journal of Library Administration,* 2, 43-65.

Matheson, N.W. and Cooper, J.A.D. (1982) Academic information in the academic health sciences center: roles for the library in information management. *Journal of Medical Education,* **57,** (10) part 2, 1-93.

Matheson, N.W., et al. (1990) Johns Hopkins University, Welsh Medical Library; in: *Campus strategies for libraries and electronic information,* edited by C.R. Arms. Bedford, MA: Digital Press. pp. 274-304

Parston, G., ed. (1987) *Managers as strategists: health services managers reflect on practice.* Ottawa, Ont.: Canadian Hospital Association.

Sheldon, B.E. (1989) Strategic planning for public library services in the 21st century. *Journal of Library Administration,* **11,** 199-208.

Swisher, R. and McClure, C.R. (1984) *Research for decision making: methods for librarians.* Chicago, Ill.: American Library Association.

Tenets, Mission, Principles, Process. (1990) Hamilton, Ont.: Faculty of Health Sciences, McMaster University, 1990.

Setting standards for quality assurance: the Canadian experience

Jan Greenwood
Manager of Corporate Records and Library Services,
Ontario Medical Association, Toronto, Ontario, Canada

Introduction

In Canada the quality assurance (QA) watchdog for health care facilities is the Canadian Council on Health Facilities Accreditation (CCHFA). The CCHFA, loved and loathed in ever-varying proportions by health professionals, is responsible for developing standards against which facilities are measured and, if successful, awarded accreditation for one, two or three years.

The accreditation programme is voluntary and independent of government. Before being surveyed each health facility must meet eligibility criteria and complete a self-evaluation process, both of which are established by the CCHFA. Accreditation survey teams include only health administrators, physicians and nurses, but a committee comprising representatives of other health professional groups ensures, at least in theory, that standards reflect the experience, needs and concerns of all health professionals. Unfortunately, for many years, the hospital library community failed to participate in the accreditation process despite the fact that Staff Library Services became a prerequisite for accreditation in 1967. The early history of hospital library standards, up to and including publication of the *Canadian Standards for Hospital Libraries* (1975) and the adoption of its descriptive recommendations by the accrediting body in 1977, has been well documented (Eagleton 1988; Flower 1978; Greenwood 1987) and will not be discussed here. It was only after the establishment of a Task Force on Hospital Library Standards by the Canadian Health Libraries Association (CHLA) in November 1986 that a concerted effort was made to re-establish a formal link between the profession and the Canadian Council on Hospital Accreditation (CCHA) as the Council was named until 1987.

Since 1983 the concept of QA has been the cornerstone of the accreditation program. It has its roots in the United States where a growing consumer advocacy movement indirectly prompted the development of hospital-wide QA monitoring and risk management programs. As Van Wyck (1985) and others have noted, however, various types of performance appraisal had been in existence in health-care organizations for years before the onslaught of QA. What changed, however, was the requirement for more formal co-ordination of these activities and the need to come to grips with a new and baffling terminology.

In the 1983 *Standards for Accreditation of Canadian Health Care Facilities* the CCHA stated unequivocally that "The health care facility's quality assurance program shall be emphasized in determining the accreditation of the facility" (CCHA 1983, 46) and, indeed, gave health facilities just three years to comply if they were to be granted full accreditation. "Quality assurance" was defined in the glossary as:

> "The program and mechanisms including clinical appraisal and utilization review which are designed to optimize the results of therapy in the constraints of the available resources both human and material." (CCHA, 1983: xx)

If this definition appears restrictive, the intent was by no means to confine QA activities to the front-line departments. In addition to a set of standards for an institution-wide QA program, were complementary standards for each accredited service, e.g. "There shall be procedures established to evaluate the quality of Library Services and performance of personnel" (CCHA, 1983: 130). It is true that this instruction was followed by standards which did not seem to measure, in any meaningful way, professional library services:

> "Records should be kept of the type and volume of periodicals, textbooks etc. that are being used as well as requests from staff or acquisitions." (CCHA, 1983: 130)

What was important, however, in this tentative foray into the world of QA was that libraries were, by implication, to be considered an integral component in a health-care institution's overall efforts to ensure optimal patient care.

Notwithstanding the issue of QA and the shockwaves that permeated small institutions in particular (Lynch, 1987, 29), the standards for library services did not meet with universal approval from health librarians in Canada. Kirchner lamented that standards for the training of library staff were ludicrous given the geographical realities of Canada, that the recommendations for the composition of library advisory committees made no mention of the librarian and, in particular, that the 1977 principle that libraries be line departments directly responsible to the administration had been omitted (Kirchner, 1983: 101–103). For Kirchner the CCHA 1983 standards were a definite disappointment.

Another reason the 1983 standards for Library Services were a disappointment from the perspective of the whole hospital library community was undoubtedly the CCHA's apparent intransigence in continually refusing to incorporate into its standards the quantitative guidelines of the 1975 *Canadian Standards for Hospital Libraries.* What hospital librarians failed to understand, largely because of the lack of formal communication between the profession and the CCHA, was the very purpose and nature of the accreditation standards. Above all, the CCHA standards were, and continue to be, generic to the extent that they are formulated to address the needs of every accredited service. In 1983 there were 24 accredited services grouped into four classes: Essential Elements, Diagnostic and Therapeutic Elements, Support Elements (into which category Library Services fall), and Special Care Services. In other words, there are relatively few variations in the wording, and none in the format, of each set of standards, irrespective of the service to which they apply.

It is a reflection of the times that hospital librarians continued, during the Task Force's deliberations, and in spite of entrenched QA programs, to press for quantitative standards rather than ones that could measure outcome. Their concerns were driven by a need to protect budgets, collections, space and staff in the face of an economic squeeze that threatened all of these in many institutions. The sheer demand placed upon library services seemed enough to justify their existence and the very idea of developing standards for measuring outcome posed a challenge for which there was neither time nor energy. Furthermore, the accreditation standards had never purported to provide measures for anything other than structure and process, and the mandate of the Task Force remained unequivocally to develop standards that could be absorbed into the CCHA framework. All of this is not to deny, however, that many health librarians were making sporadic attempts within their own QA programmes to assess user satisfaction with specific services by means of user surveys and other mechanisms.

Development of the Standards for Canadian Health Care Facility Libraries, 1989

With full recognition of the constraints imposed by the generic standards of CCHA the Task Force set about establishing terms of reference (Greenwood, 1989: 2-3). Initially the CHLA Board had given the Task Force a mandate to revise the 1975 *Canadian Standards for Hospital Libraries.* However, it appeared very early in the process that what would be more acceptable would be a revision of the CCHA 1986 edition of its standards for Library Services. The reason for this decision was that any descriptive standards developed by CHLA appeared more likely to be incorporated into those of the CCHA if they were to conform in format and wording to the generic document. At that time also the Task Force was as concerned about educating accreditation surveyors and health facility administrators as it was interested in providing health librarians with working standards by which their services could reasonably be measured. This mission shaped, in large measure, the document which was finally published in 1989 and endorsed by the CHLA Board as the professional practice guidelines or standards for health facility libraries in Canada (CHLA, 1989).

Thus, these professional standards include not only a set of descriptive standards modelled on those published by the CCHA, up to and including the 1986 edition, but also complementary qualitative and quantitative guidelines, an interpretation for small health care facilities, a glossary and bibliography, and a "Form for Assessing the Quality of Libraries in Health Care Facilities".

The decision to base a set of descriptive standards upon the CCHA 1986 edition led to the development of standards relating to each of the following:

1. Goals and Objectives

2. Organization and Administration

3. Direction and Staffing

4. Facilities, Equipment and Supplies

5. Policies and Procedures

6. Information Resources and Services

7. Education

8. Quality Assurance

With one exception the organization of these standards conforms exactly to the CCHA version, although the content of each has been greatly expanded and the emphasis changed to reflect current library practices. Also, the principle for Library Services, that they "shall be maintained for all of the professional and auxiliary staff as appropriate" (CCHA, 1986: 147), was replaced by a mission statement which could readily be adapted for use in facilities of all sizes and complexity:

> "Library Services shall be organized and administered to meet the information needs of all hospital and medical staff, students, patients and affiliated health professionals in support of patient care, education, management, research and outreach services consistent with the mission statement of the health-care facility." CHLA, 1989: 10)

This mission statement, like any mission statement, cannot be used to measure the value of the services being provided, but it does at least specify who should be served and for what purposes. This is important for Canadian health facility libraries because they have been granted through accreditation at least as broad a mandate as any other hospital department and many have suffered in recent times from reporting to services with narrower, and therefore conflicting mandates. Although few Canadian health facility libraries have an official mandate (or resources) to serve patient and consumer health information needs, the Task Force chose to include service to patients because many libraries are, in practice, providing these services and this trend is likely to gain momentum as hospitals appeal more and more to their local communities for funding to supplement or match government grants.

Standard I: Goals and Objectives.

Health facility librarians were disquieted by the 1986 standards for goals and objectives that appeared to give hospital administrators too much leeway for interpretation: "The extent and scope of library services ... will

vary with the size and responsibilities of the facility. " (CCHA, 1986: 177)
To counteract the vagueness necessitated by the generic formula the Task
Force introduced a standard requiring that goals and objectives for library
services be developed by professional librarians. The remaining standards
under "Goals and Objectives" in the CHLA document require simply that
there be goals and objectives for each of the issues addressed by the other
seven standards: staffing, physical facility, collection, access to information,
co-operative arrangements with other libraries, equipment, continuing education and QA.

Standard II: Organization and Administration.

Within this standard the Task Force took the opportunity to reinstate the
pre-1983 accreditation requirement that Library Services be organized as a
separate department reporting directly to the administration. The ramifi-
cations of this recommendation continue to reverberate unsatisfactorily in
1990 as the CCHFA 1991 standards go to press. The issue of satellite or
departmental libraries in health facilities is one which seems to plague hospital librarians everywhere. Standard I addresses this issue by stating that
"the principal information resources of the health-care facility collections
shall be housed in the central library"; that "Departmental collections shall
be limited to those information resources necessary to the daily function-
ing of the given department"; and, lastly, that "the library shall maintain
a central catalogue of all information resources owned by the health care
facility and facilitate access to them." (CHLA, 1989: 11) An introductory
standard requires that: "the library staff shall be responsible for developing
a cost-effective acquisitions program for obtaining the health-care facility's
information resources" (CHLA, 1989: 11)

  Although there was controversy in the field about the value of library advisory committees, the Task Force chose to retain the relevant standards. In
particular, the Task Force felt that advisory committees might have an important role to play in identifying new programmes and services that could,
potentially, have an impact on library services, but which might otherwise
not come to the attention of the librarian during the critical planning phase.

Standard III: Direction and Staffing.

Of all the contentious issues the Task Force faced, this was the one that
proved to be the most challenging. At the root of the problem were the con-

flicting needs of having professional involvement in all library services, and the impossibility of hiring a professional librarian in every health care facility, no matter how small. Ultimately a compromise was reached by allowing the concept of direction by a professional librarian to include consultative services in one form or another:

> "All library services shall be directed by a qualified professional librarian on a full-time, part-time, or continuing consultative basis consonant with the needs of the health care facility." (CHLA, 1989: 12)

The CHLA standards for "Direction and Staffing" also differ significantly from the CCHA 1986 edition by recognizing the need for various levels of expertise in libraries, i.e. professional, technical and clerical. Many small health libraries in Canada are maintained by library technicians or clerical staff and the Task Force was as keen to prevent library technicians from being inappropriately usurped by untrained staff as it was to ensure that every library service benefited from professional direction. It is in the matter of staffing that the CHLA Task Force has made some of its most significant gains in terms of the proposed CCHFA standards for 1991.

Standard IV: Facilities, Equipment and Supplies.

This set of CHLA standards improves upon the CCHA generic document by dragging the health facility library into the technological age. Standards address the obvious technological issues of online services, computer-assisted instruction and end-user searching, as well as recognizing the need for space to accommodate varied user activities. The accreditation standards of 1986 pay little attention to staff needs and do not contain any standards for the space required by users; spacial requirements for staff workspace are limited to "acquisition, cataloguing, typing, filing, processing new material" and the "preparation of volumes for binding." (CCHA, 1986: 148)

Standard V: Policies and Procedures.

Every Canadian hospital librarian knows that even the most cursory examination of library services by the accreditation surveyors will entail a request for the departmental policies and procedures manual. To this end the CHLA descriptive standards require that policies and procedures shall relate to an extensive and varied list of issues, ranging from the formulation of goals and objectives through professional ethics and collection maintenance to QA programmes and staff development (CHLA, 1989: 14)

Standard VI: Information Resources and Services.

The most significant difference between the CHLA descriptive standards and the CCHA generic document upon which they were based is the introduction of a set of standards for Information Resources and Services. These standards were designed to correspond to the CCHA "Care Program" standards which were intended to provide measures for success in evaluating professional, direct, patient-care services. The 1986 standards did not include an equivalent standard for Library Services and, as a result, the professional responsibilities of libraries were, at best, diffused among the standards for "Organization and Administration", "Direction and Staffing" and "Policies and Procedures" and, at worst, omitted altogether. The lack of standards for professional library services inevitably led to a disproportionate emphasis being placed upon non-professional tasks.

Standards VII and VIII: Education and Quality Assurance.

Given that the standards pertaining to education and QA are essentially generic, the Task Force made few amendments other than to include a standard under the former requiring that "particular attention shall be paid to programs relating to changing information technology." (CHLA, 1989: 16)

Qualitative Guidelines

For each set of descriptive standards described above the CHLA document provides qualitative guidelines which were developed as an educational tool for health administrators, as well as for practical use by librarians. The guidelines include sample terms of reference for library advisory committees, definitions of various levels of library staff, a brief guide to physical planning, sample outlines for a general policies and procedures manual and one for collection development, and some sample library audits.

Quantitative Guidelines

The quantitative guidelines were derived from published sources, such as the *Canadian Standards for Hospital Libraries* (1975), the *New York Standards*

(University of the State of New York, 1983) and the Medical Library Association's *Minimum Standards* ... (1984), and also from data obtained from
two questionnaires which the Task Force distributed to every CHLA hospital
library member. Thus do these guidelines simultaneously reflect and direct
current library practices in Canadian health facilities.

Recognizing that changing patterns of health-care delivery have had a
dramatic impact upon library services since publication of the *Canadian
Standards for Hospital Libraries* in 1975, the Task Force decided to review
carefully the characteristics that were chosen to categorize hospitals 12 years
earlier. In addition to the number of beds, affiliation with a medical school,
accreditation for internship and residency, research commitment and numbers of staff, which had all been indicators for classification of facilities in
the 1975 document, the Task Force added for assessment the number of ad-
missions, ambulatory care or emergency care visits, referral centre responsibilities and libraries serving multi-institutional systems. On the basis of
these indicators the CHLA document defines four health facility categories,
A through D in descending order of size and complexity, and provides an
"Interpretation for Small Health Facilities" in what amounts to a fifth category.

The core list of minimum user services for libraries in the four categories, A through D, comprises: online search services (external access only
for Category D institutions), manual searches of printed indexes (excluding
Category A), orientation to library services and resources, provision of information, convenient access to photocopy facilities, interlibrary loans, acquisitions lists, verification of reference citations and co-ordination of the facility's
bibliographic and audiovisual resources. Recommendations for Categories A
and B also include MEDLINE on CD-ROM, bibliographic instruction, user
education on storing, accessing and retrieving electronic information, current awareness services, document delivery, end-user support and referral
or specialized services. "Additional recommended services" for category A
institutions are: clinical health librarian programme, patient education and
consumer health information services, training for library students, exhibits
in library and an index to research in progress in the health care facility.

For each institutional category the CHLA document includes specific staff
quotas, recommending also professional, technical and clerical ratios. Similarly, minimum numerical requirements for books and journals are given with
retention guidelines for the latter. Because the use of audiovisual resources
and equipment varies so much among Canadian health-care institutions the
Task Force chose to make only a broad recommendation that audiovisual

resources and services "support affiliated teaching programmes and health care facility in-service and continuing education".

As no usable formula was available for determining library budgets, and given that the Task Force recommendation that all libraries be directed by a professional library permeates the entire document, the following statement was deemed to suffice for all categories:

> "The budget shall be adequate to cover all user services, staff salaries and continuing education, resources, including audiovisual and computer software, technology, equipment and any co-operative arrangements." (CHLA, 1989)

In making recommendations for physical space the Task Force opted for a modular approach to allow flexibility and interpretation by libraries in every institutional category: e.g. seating space for 10% of primary users and 1% of secondary users; 225 square feet per computer workstation; standard library shelving allowing 4.5–5 journal volumes and 7–8 books per linear foot. Guidelines for live-load, lighting, temperature and humidity requirements are also provided.

Assessment Form

To enable health facility libraries to carry out an overall audit of their services the Task Force developed a "Form for assessing the Quality of Libraries in Health Care Facilities". although the New York standards (University of New York, 1983) provided the prototype, substantial changes were made to ensure that the rating for libraries in each institutional category corresponded accurately with the descriptive, qualitative and quantitative standards.

CCHFA Standards revision project

The CCHFA announcement in 1988 that it was embarking on a 2-year project to overhaul radically the accreditation process, as well as the format of the complementary documents, was a mixed blessing for the Task Force. It was clear that the completed descriptive standards which had been based upon the CCHA 1986 documents could not be re-written, and therefore would likely bear little resemblance to any new accreditation standards. However, health librarians were now in the enviable position of having a comprehensive set of standards that reflected current practices and might be used to influence the content of the new accreditation standards even if they were at variance in format.

The mechanism for influencing the CCHFA lay in the establishment of a National Organizations Committee in which approximately 30 professional associations and other organizations were invited to participate. While, in theory, this is an excellent vehicle for encouraging the participation of the professions governed by the accreditation standards, in fact most of the cards are in the hands of the CCHFA and the mechanism has proved to be flawed in large measure by virtue of each organization dealing in isolation with its own set of service standards. Hampered by the admittedly enormous task, tight deadlines and, perhaps most of all, its own formulaic approach to setting standards, the CCHFA is not always rigorous in communicating to its National Organization representatives generic (across the board) changes to various standards and sometimes does not appear to have an understanding of how significant could be the impact of some of these on certain services. Because the deadlines given to the representatives to review the various drafts are often totally unrealistic — days rather than weeks in some cases — it is easy to miss small but critical variations in the wording of documents that, to all intents and purposes, appear identical.

In spite of these serious impediments to the process, and a number of extremely disappointing (and unilateral) decisions by CCHFA with respect to the wording, the standards for Library Services approved for implementation in 1991 show a marked improvement over their predecessors (CCHFA, 1990). To a greater extent than might have been thought possible they have incorporated much of the spirit and content of the CHLA descriptive standards, with one notable exception. Unfortunately the greatest concern to health librarians, which was the need to report to a department with a compatible mandate, is not addressed in the new standards. On the grounds that it cannot interfere with the organizational autonomy of individual health facilities, the CCHFA has chosen instead a generic statement that "the appropriate authority may be: ...the next level of management responsible for the service" (CCHFA, 1990: 12). However, the functions attributed to Library Services under Standard I, Statement of Purpose, Goals and Objectives, previously comprising mainly non-professional tasks, now correspond almost precisely to the recommendations of CHLA (CCHFA, 1990, 1). With respect to staffing, the CCHFA has finally introduced a standard that requires of health librarians ("directors of the service") appropriate educational qualifications and, further, for the first time makes explicit their managerial responsibilities by citing 12 managerial accountabilities which also apply to each of the other services (CCHFA, 1990, 8).

The CCHFA is intent upon developing standards for the nineties that will place new emphasis upon outcome measures and risk management and is thus currently involved in an outcome measures project on the quality of care. Andersen, in reporting upon a recent national conference on risk management involving CCHFA, describes the concept as management philosophy that depends, for its institutional success, "on a reduction of loss through QA, high-quality care and effective resource utilization" (1990: 40). However, as we have seen, what has emerged so far from CCHFA are standards that remain unequivocally descriptive and generic. Bilodeau, speaking of QA programmes in general, goes so far as to say that "Our problem is that we have no way of measuring quality of care, and neither does the Canadian Council of Health Facilities Accreditation." (1989: 10) Although the 1990 CCHFA document refers repeatedly to the concepts of risk management and utilization review, the responsibility for developing relevant standards is left to the individual accredited services. One or two examples might serve to clarify the way in which CCHFA is approaching these thorny issues. One of the 12 managerial accountabilities alluded to above is: "conducting or guiding quality assurance, utilization review and risk management activities." (CCHFA, 1990: 8) Similarly Standard II stipulates that there shall be policies and procedures for risk management and utilization review (CCHFA, 1990: 10), while another standard ensures that there are mechanisms for the participation of all service directors in any facility-wide activities pertaining to these (CCHFA, 1990: 6).

Interestingly, just as the pressure mounts to develop better standards or outcome measures, QA as an accredited, institution-wide programme is being withdrawn from the CCHFA standards. The responsibility for all QA activities is, therefore, now squarely placed upon the shoulders of the individual services. This move will provide both a challenge and an opportunity for health librarians. As far back as 1987, when QA was still a relatively new phenomenon in Canada, one librarian astutely noted that QA was in danger of becoming a substitute for professional judgement (Smithies, 1987: 147). Clemenhagen echoes this sentiment in writing that "Practitioners are the only ones truly able to cut QA bureaucracy and define meaningful quality assurance activities" (1987: 9). Even in 1987 there would have been library cynics who could identify with O'Brien's sense that there was disillusionment with the QA process among health professionals in general, and would not have been surprised to hear of an increase in patient dissatisfaction, as well as a rise in the number of lawsuits against health facilities, in spite of the established programmes (1987: 22).

In 1990 the current standards of both CHLA and CCHFA remain, at face value, no more than rather crude measures of input. They certainly are a long way from answering the question of whether, let alone how satisfactorily, hospital libraries are having an impact upon the quality of patient care. McFarlane's contention in 1985 that there were no ready-made standards by which to measure what ought to be achieved remains valid (McFarlane, 1985, 184), and there is no question that health librarians will soon have to grapple with the difficult task of developing standards that measure user satisfaction with library services, but it is a moot point whether any standards for libraries could really be used as a measure of patient care outcomes. One may, of course, count how many books are catalogued within an hour or interlibrary loans processed in a day, and even develop a standard for performance within a given library or for libraries in general, but how does one ensure that their being catalogued or processed (however quickly and meticulously) actually contributes to the quality of patient care? Could standards ever be developed to ensure, for example, that any information provided is used intelligently and effectively? Gillespie, who developed one of the first comprehensive QA programmes in health libraries in Canada, implicitly hit the nail on the head when she defined QA as follows:

> "Quite simply, a quality assurance program is a management tool which uses formal monitoring techniques to identify and assess the quality of a product. In the health-care setting, the product is the care and service provided to patients; in libraries quality assurance measures the service provided to users and the procedures which provide the service." (Gillespie, 1985: 187)

There we have the rub; health libraries, perhaps with the exception of those incorporating clinical medical librarian programs, remain irretrievably one step removed from what must be the focus of all facility-wide QA programmes, the patient.

Conclusion

All of this does not mean, of course, that health libraries are not valuable or, because their services cannot easily be evaluated within the widely accepted

QA framework, that health librarians should feel defeated by the established process. Nor does it mean that standards do not have a role to play in determining the quality of library services. There is unquestionably a great deal of informal evidence that libraries are fully worth their expense (Hardy et al., 1985: 46); a fact that has not been lost on the medical community. A spokesperson for the Medical Society of the State of New York recently delivered a scathing rebuke to the State's Department of Health for eliminating a minimum standard requiring hospitals to maintain a library to be eligible for federal funding, concluding that "The loss of hospital medical libraries will adversely impact (sic) on the quality of care .... " (Farnsworth, 1989: 602) Certainly, during the last decade, the Ontario Medical Association's (OMA) Consulting Library Service has responded to literally hundreds of requests from physicians and allied health professionals to assist in improving libraries in their institutions, and there is mounting evidence to suggest that rural hospitals, in particular, are under pressure to upgrade their libraries to meet existing standards because of difficulties encountered in hiring today's graduates who are unwilling to settle for rudimentary information services (Greenwood, consulting files). Furthermore the OMA files reveal a high degree of satisfaction among users of health facility libraries in response to service-specific questionnaires.

Even in the face of trends toward outcome measures, risk management and utilization review it seems unlikely that the limitations that have beset standards to date — their focus upon inputs and disregard for the unique characteristics which differentiate individual libraries from one another — will disappear completely. But standards remain valuable because, as Duchow states, they represent "the aggregate experience of the professionals and experts behind them." (1985: 179) After all, without sound inputs, how can any library expect to deliver optimum service? Standards will remain an important stepping stone in the ceaseless march toward excellence; they will continue to present embryonic libraries with a framework for development, and will provide important political ammunition for the continued support of those that have already achieved excellence. Standards, by themselves, will not prove that support services have a direct and positive effect on the quality of patient care. Professional librarians will, however, continue to use them in conjunction with other mechanisms for measuring user satisfaction with library services. Beyond that they will have to rise to a new challenge: that of engaging in research to establish the vital link between information services and the provision of high quality patient care. The King study (1987) gives one every reason for optimism that the results will prove conclusively that good library services are an essential component in this endeavour.

References

Andersen, H. B. A. (1990) Risk management comes of age. *Dimensions,* **67**, (1), 40–41.

Bilodeau, M. (1989) Quality indicators should emphasize outcomes. *Dimensions,* **66** (3), 9–10.

Canadian Council on Health Facilities Accreditation. (1990) *Library services: long term care facilities.* [Unpublished document approved for forthcoming publication of 1991 standards for Canadian acute and long term care facilities (in press).]

Canadian Council on Hospital Accreditation. (1983) *Guide to accreditation of Canadian health-care facilities.* Ottawa: CCHA.

Canadian Council on Hospital Accreditation. (1986) *Guide to accreditation of Canadian health-care facilities.* Ottawa: CCHA.

Canadian standards for hospital libraries. (1975) *Canadian Medical Association Journal,* **112**, 1271–1274.

Clemenhagen, C. (1987) Overcoming the barriers to QA. *Dimensions* **64** (8), 6,9.

Duchow, S. R. (1985) Quality assurance for health and hospital libraries: general considerations and background. *Bibliotheca Medica Canadiana,* **6**, 177–181.

Eagleton, K. M. (1988) Quality assurance in Canadian hospital libraries – the challenge of the eighties. *Health Libraries Review,* **5**, (3), 145–154.

Farnsworth, P. B. (1989) The elemination of the requirement for medical libraries in hospitals. *New York State Journal of Medicine,* **89**, 601–602.

Flower, M.A. (1978) Toward hospital library standards in Canada. *Bulletin of the Medical Libraries Association,* **66**, 296–301.

Gillespie, S. A. (1985) QA do's and don'ts: or points to consider when designing a library quality assurance program. *Bibliotheca Medica Canadiana,* **6**, 187–191.

Greenwood, J. (1987) Standards for medical and health care libraries: Canada. *Inspel,* **21**, (4), 24–31.

Greenwood, J. (1989) *Introduction. Standards for Canadian health care facility libraries: qualitative and quantitative guidelines for assessment.* Toronto: CHLA, 1989.

Hardy, M. C., Yeoh, J. W. and Crawford, S. (1985) Evaluating the impact of library services on the quality and cost of medical care. *Bulletin of the Medical Libraries Association,* **73**, 43–46.

King, D. N. (1987) The contribution of hospital library information services to clinical care: a study in eight hospitals. *Bulletin of the Medical Libraries Association,* **75**, 291–301.

Kirchner, A. K. (1983) Standards and hospital libraries: observations on the 1983 edition of the Canadian Council on hospital Accreditation, standards for accreditation of Canadian health care facilities — library services. *Bibliotheca Medica Canadiana,* **5**, 101–103.

Lynch, J. F. (1987) Quality assurance in the small health care facility. *Dimensions,* **64**, (4), 29–32.

McFarlane, L. (1985) QA: a personal perspective. *Bibliotheca Medica Canadiana,* **6**, 182–185.

Medical Library Association. (1984) *Minimum standards for health sciences libraries in hospitals.* Chicago: MLA.

O'Brien, N., Lowe, C. and Rennebohm, H. (1987) A managerial perspective on controlling the quality of patient care. *Dimensions,* **64**, (4), 22–23,26–28.

Smithies, R. (1985) Quality assurance in the health sciences library. *Bibliotheca Medica Canadiana,* **6**, 146–147.

University of the State of New York. (1983) *Manual for assessing the quality of health sciences libraries in hospitals.* Albany, NY: State University of New York.

Van Wyck, P. (1985) An administrative overview of quality assurance. *Bibliotheca Medica Canadiana,* **6**, 141–145.

Setting standards for quality assurance: the European Experience

Fiona Mackay Picken
Regional Librarian, NW Thames Regional Library and
Information Service and British Postgraduate Medical
Federation, University of London, U.K.

Introduction

> "Cross-national enquiry into organization and management is a
> particularly arduous field of investigation but the question re-
> mains whether we can afford to ignore it in our increasingly
> inter-dependent and international world" (Child 1981, quoted
> by Magalhães 1985).

It should be added that investigations in Europe are especially complex
as twenty-one languages are involved. Many words do not translate neatly or
exactly into other languages, which results in distortion of meaning. This can
lead to imprecision and confusion, especially in the field of standards where
the language of genesis is American English, whereas traditionally most Eu-
ropeans learn standard English. The additional dimension of re-translation
involving three languages increases the possibility of misunderstanding.

The setting of standards is a field of growing importance as witnessed
by the increasing number of publications in the U.K. alone (DHSS 1970, Library Association 1978, Council for Postgraduate Medical Education 1981,
NHS/DHSS Health Service Information Steering Group 1985, General Medical Council 1987, DHSS 1989, King's Fund Centre 1990). It is also an area

which now provokes much interest and, in the course of my enquiries, it emerged that other people's published standards are greatly desired and are clearly regarded by some as a solution to local and national problems.

Against the patchwork of European languages should be set the rich diversity of culture, history and attitudes. Given this background, it seems unlikely that, in the foreseeable future, Europe will evolve one set of standards for medical and health libraries. On the other hand, by making existing standards available, other countries can establish appropriate measures relevant to their national situation, while developing their own. To what extent there is scope for an overall European umbrella set, with national subsets to accommodate local variants, remains to be seen.

Data collection for this study

Europe was a very dynamic area during the 1980s; partly because the European Community (EC) gave great impetus to co-operative ventures and this stimulated even countries which are not formal members of the EC to participate in activities of mutual benefit and interest. The European Association of Health Information & Libraries (EAHIL) was founded in 1986 and its activities have been constrained only by the lack of time and money of its members. Its membership list, coupled with personal acquaintance provided one initial contact point per country. Twenty-five countries were contacted in September 1989. By June 1990 replies had been received from 21: the remaining four were mainly relatively small countries which were unlikely to formulate their own standards, or Central and East European countries caught up in the political turmoils of late 1989.

It is due to the willing co-operation of these countries that this paper is possible, as the personal knowledge of the respondents in referring to unpublished or Committee activity gives a very different picture to that in the published literature. To ensure that any relevant activity was identified, information was requested under the following terms: (1) Quality Assurance; (2) Health Library Standards; (3) Audit; (4) Performance Indicators; (5) Library Evaluation. This follows the pattern set by Ursula Hausen who presented a paper at the 1987 IFLA General Conference in Brighton, U.K. entitled "Standards for medical and health care libraries: Europe", upon which I have drawn for background material.

Preconditions for the development of standards

From previous observation and investigation, and from the responses to this study, it is clear that there are certain pre- conditions for the production of standards:

1. The establishment of a professional body of librarians and information scientists. Librarians themselves must realize that they are professionals, that they have to push to gain recognition, and that this will only come from valuing themselves. Self-value, self-respect and self-confidence are essential (Magalhães 1952, Picken 1979). The formation and development of a professional organization is essential. No individual can create a standard.

2. The establishment of library and information science schools. The formal recognition that literature and information handling require special skills brings about the establishing of formal qualifications, which in turn provide levers for status and acceptance. Peer group pressure between professions is crucial and equal recognition will give documents produced by professional bodies status and authority.

3. Gathering statistics, analysing them and using the results.

4. Conducting surveys, analysing the results and using the evidence so acquired.

5. Setting up pilot studies and amending the protocol in the light of results.

All the foregoing form part of an infrastructure on which to build. It is essential that there be a solid basis for extrapolation and that standards reflect a sense of reality.

Just as there are preconditions for the development of standards, there is a common thread of reasons for the failure to formulate or apply standards. The main reason is the adoption of overambitious aims. The setting of impossible targets such as proposing very large budgets or generous staffing levels which are out of balance with related fields is not helpful and can lead to the work being dismissed out of hand.

Strategies

So far, it can be seen that setting standards for quality assurance in relation to medical and health libraries is an accretive process. Fully fledged standards are arrived at gradually. Newcomers often express surprise at the lack of standards in a field established for hundreds of years, and where it would seem that they would have a beneficial effect. Those who have worked on this would agree — in principle. The obstacles, however, only assume their intransigence in the course of detailed discussions and projections. Standards have to be a consensus view. But, should they try to strike a balance between the bare minimum and the unattainably high? Should they set an example and state what is really needed? Or should they begin as a minimum and gradually work towards a more elevated target with revisions building on achievement? The problem with the continuous approach is the continuous commitment. Most people who care about standards are already very active in their field generally. If they finally succeed in persuading hundreds of colleagues to agree to whatever imperfect document is produced, it is depressing to think the revision process starts there.

Acceptance of a published set of standards is fundamental. One of the reasons why the UK Library Association Guidelines for Library Provision in the Health Service (Library Association, 1978) have not been widely used, is that the figures lacked reality. It cannot be re-iterated too often that a) credibility is a key feature and b) standards are neither immutable nor eternal and that regular revisions are an integral part of the process.

The foregoing could seem rather negative, so a few strategies for self-help will be discussed. Referring back to the accretive nature of standards, it is possible, with a certain amount of skill and lateral thinking, to make deductions and draw conclusions from any set of comparable figures. For example, if you get figures covering the same activities from even two libraries, simple addition and division will give you an average. Do this with ten or twenty and you can start to determine patterns and the resulting figures will tell you a considerable amount. If you are familiar with the respondents and can put in caveats or put a gloss or weighting on the final results this will render them even more useful. On the other hand, it is perfectly possible for someone with no inside knowledge to do an analysis of given sets of figures and reach certain conclusions.

Anyone can do this at any time. A librarian should keep figures of all activity from the day of appointment. By analysing queries received, or interlibrary loans requested/fulfilled, week against week, month against month, year against year, patterns appear, averages are determined, marked increases or decreases detected. If these can be demonstrated graphically it is even more effective. A graph with a dramatically rising line can be a more powerful ally than a dozen reports, and can convince even the most hardened administrator. Everyone can monitor his or her activity and acquire valuable information, but this is also the raw data on which wider studies will be built and no one should hesitate to impose this small self-discipline.

To demonstrate more precisely what can be done, a paper on a survey of Turkish Medical School Libraries (Brennan, et al., 1987) was analysed in this way. The following example shows how any set of comparable figures can be used, and how a league table may be derived from them. The resulting average or standard can then be used as the starting point for comparisons.

University	Volumes	Journals	Budget	Staff
1 Cukorova	45,000	N/A	204,166	18
2 Ankara	20,132	301	39,583	11
3 Hacettepe	90,000	750	135,416	36
4 Gazi	3,500	270	75,000	14
5 Akdeniz	3,150	69	6,250	2
6 Uludag	25,000	181	14,583	4
7 Dicle	20,200	85	20,833	9
8 Anadolu	13,000	60	27,083	3
9 Istanbul-1	55,119	208	15,625	19
10 Istanbul-2	40,009	206	15,625	14

Table 1: Characteristics of Turkish medical school libraries

If one then uses the staff element as the yardstick, one can calculate each element "handled" per staff member, as shown in Table 2, which shows that the average Turkish medical school library has 13 staff and that each member of staff relates to 2690 volumes, 22 current journals and 4380 units of budget.

This permits scaling up or down, or even laterally, so that, if you have four staff, to achieve parity with the average you should have 10,760 volumes, 88 journal titles and a budget of 17,520.

To achieve parity with the average for Turkey: 9 staff are needed to manage 25,000 volumes, and 8 staff are needed to manage 181 journals, but to manage a budget of 14,583 would require only 3 staff. If, therefore, you do have 8 staff, your budget should be 35,000 units.

Library	Staff nos.	Volumes	Journals	Budget
Lib 1	18	2500	N/A	11,340
Lib 2	11	1830	27	3,636
Lib 3	36	2500	21	3,761
Lib 4	14	250	19	5,357
Lib 5	2	1575	34	3,125
Lib 6	4	6250	45	3,645
Lib 7	9	2244	9	2,314
Lib 8	3	4333	20	9,000
Lib 9	19	2901	11	822
Lib 10	14	2857	19	1,116

Table 2: Number of items/staff in Turkish medical school libraries.

Thus, the averages are: 13 staff, 2690 volumes, 22 journals and 4,380 units of budget.

It must be emphasised that this is an academic exercise. It in no way recommends that Turkish medical libraries should be staffed and stocked or funded in this way. This is simply to demonstrate that figures are a vital element in devising standards and can be used very effectively as a starting point. Those below average can agitate for parity with the norm. Those above average can congratulate themselves, while considering whether the results reflect desirable balances.

A crude measure which I have used is based on the fact that UK acute general hospitals have comparable staffing levels which are based on bed numbers: i.e., any 500 bedded hospital, has X doctors, Y nurses, Z administrators, and N nurses, and these are the users to whom a service is offered. By taking the revenue (recurrent) budget of the library and dividing it into the number of beds in the on-site hospital, one gets a league table. Within the National Health Service (NHS) District General Hospitals are on the same financial footing, all have basically the same objectives and all have the same source of funding: their Regional Health Authority.

These figures have proved to be very effective in the NHS as they are readily understood by both doctors and administrators and they demonstrate relative positions in a pointed manner. So far libraries at the bottom of the league table have never failed to get (relatively) substantial injections of funds by using these standards in making cases. By combining with colleagues and working out what one wants to attain, steps can be taken to develop parameters which will determine not only what needs to be collected, but what can be achieved with the figures afterwards.

The staged approach is realistic, as it harnesses and organises figures most probably already collected or at least available, and builds on them. From these beginnings, projections can be made and objectives shifted from struggling up from the bottom to the average, to trying to become one of the leaders. In the meantime of course, the average is automatically shifting as the poorest make up lost ground. This has been proved in my NHS Region, by a change is costs (excluding salaries) from £13.50 per bed in 1986 to £27.52 in 1989. The cost of books and journals has increased by approximately 30–40% during those three years, but the expenditure per bed has increased by over 100

Overview of European position on standards

The data collection exercise described earlier provides the following picture of standards in Greater Europe in mid 1990.

1. Comprehensive standards.

Apart from the Institute for Scientific Information in Medicine in the German Democratic Republic (Hausen 1987), no fully prescribed standards seem to be in operation in Europe. Hausen cites Standards for Dutch medical libraries in general hospitals published in 1987 but I have found nothing as to their effect.

2. Organisations.

The formation of biomedical library groups seems to be gaining ground, as well as the work done by existing organisations. For example, in Greece, the Union of Greek Libraries, has re-convened a Committee of Standards for Special Libraries, including medical libraries. Official standards have already been produced such as "Title page of a book" (Standard 676); "Library catalogue card dimensions" (Standard 367, 1979); "Abstracts in serial publications" (Standard 720, 1982). Denmark has had the Library Research Council for many years, which has done valuable work on library design and equipment, but has not involved itself specifically in biomedical libraries. Switzerland has the more general Association of Swiss Librarians (ASL) and the Committee of Biomedical Libraries. The latter has formulated qualitative standards such as a 24 hour handling process for document delivery by medical schools. It has also issued standards on subject cataloguing by MeSH and standards for the Union Catalogue of Periodicals.

In Spain, in 1989, one biomedical organisation of libraries was created by the Basques and one was established in Andalucia. An interim co-ordinating team was established with a representative from each Province within Andalucia. In the last ten years, both Portugal and Italy have formed biomedical librarian organisations. In the UK, the Medical Section of the Library Association was created after the Second World War. This has developed into the Medical Health and Welfare Libraries Group of the LA with around 1800 members. Over the years it has produced various publications which one would now refer to as standards, such as Books and Periodicals for Medical Libraries, as well as a Directory of Medical and Health Libraries in the UK.

3. Current Practice.

In some cases national bodies are using existing standards and guidelines from other countries. Greece, for example, states it is using existing European or American standards where appropriate. The Netherlands uses MeSH and the NLM classification scheme, although they are in the process of producing adaptations in Dutch (Hausen 1987).

In the UK, on the other hand, several publications over the years have been contributing to the improvement of hospital libraries. A seminal one was published by the Department of Health in 1970 called Library Services in Hospitals (G.B. Dept Health 1970). The Guidelines for Library Provision in the Health Service (Library Association, 1978), already mentioned, although much longer, were of less practical use. Amongst other things, there was confusion as to what was being recommended for patient's libraries and what was for medical libraries; the stock standards fell between the two stools of being an amalgam between medical school library requirements and hospital libraries. The result appeared to suggest extravagant resource recommendations for hospitals, but seriously inadequate provision for medical school libraries. Neither had credibility, and so they were less useful than they should have been. A very useful document on space requirements for libraries was 10 years in gestation, but in its final draft form was being used as the standard long before its publication in November 1989 (GB Dept of Health 1989). This reinforces the absolute necessity of acceptability.

4. Surveys and comparative and evaluative studies.

The survey technique is a fundamental part of the process leading to Quality Assurance(QA), consisting of assessment to determine essential elements or levels to be attained. This in turn is the basis on which a qualitative norm can be proposed. Italy has been engaged in a considerable amount of this activity, for example in Emilia-Romagna (Cavazza 1990) and Rome (Alberani 1986). France conducts user surveys, as does Spain. Ribes Cot (1990) gave a most interesting comparative paper of the users' knowledge of bibliographic tools in the medical schools, at the Bologna Conference in 1988 of the European Association of Medical and Health Libraries. The comprehensive survey of Turkish medical school libraries has many useful points (Brennan 1987), as demonstrated earlier in this paper.

Switzerland reports a sensitive salaries survey by the Association of Swiss Librarians and the UK Library Association produces an annual salary guide for various employer groups - schools, universities, the civil service, and the NHS. (Library Association, annual). This has had varying effects in different parts of the country. My own region (North-West Thames), is on the verge of accepting it as the regional standard. Staffing surveys have shown very great variations, not only throughout Europe, but within each country. These range from the observation from Cyprus that, as the sole medical librarian, he was a "one person country", not even a one-man band. Cavazza (1990) reports that in Emilia-Romagna 70% of the "librarians" in hospital libraries are administrators, not qualified librarians, of whom there are only two in post. The process of evaluation of libraries moves us nearer to quality assurance as judgement is built into library evaluation. Bulgaria, while reporting no published work on standards, specifically mentions a corpus of unpublished work on library evaluation.

5. Parallel developments.

Activity taking place in other fields should be used if relevant. In Finland, performance indicators developed for public libraries are being adapted for biomedical ones. In a separate but related field, standards relating to the education and training of the medical profession, the UK General Medical Council, specifically mentions essential facilities such as libraries (General Medical Council 1987). Incidentally, the General Medical Council is an example of absolute standards of an ethical or moral nature as well as professional competence. If medical practitioners fail to meet these stringent requirements, they are legally disbarred from practice. The Royal Colleges (of Surgeons, of Physicians, of Psychiatrists etc.) are the official regulating bodies in the UK who set and monitor through regular approval team visits, the training programmes and facilities of junior doctors in training, of which the library forms an important part.

The Royal College of Psychiatrists is especially vigilant regarding library facilities and has no compunction about refusing, or giving provisional approval only, to the doctors' entire training programme if the library is deficient. Recently too, the UK government has announced a massive programme of quality measures to be introduced generally into the NHS. These build on existing work such as the reports into maternal and peri-operative death. Programmes of audit in obstetrics, surgery, anaesthetics, and general practice are being carried out all over the country. It behoves us not only to extract from such work methods or techniques which we could develop, but also to graft qualitative aspects of library provision on to these existing activities.

6. Hindrances.

While in no way making excuses, quite a few respondents mentioned specific hindrances which prevented the development of standards and, hence, quality assurance programmes. In a fascinating paper, Magalhães (1985) examines in depth cultural factors relating to library development, and this will be taken up again later. Finland mentioned 17th century university statutes being changed. Cyprus mentions finance, ignorance of the importance of libraries, and shortage of staff. The one librarian in Cyprus was trained as recently as 1987. Cavazza (1990) too, cites the lack of recognition of the profession.

Greece has always had problems with the transliteration of the Greek alphabet, while Hausen(1987) mentions the Trades Union element in Scandinavia, as well as the recognition by the West German authorities of the fact that acceptance of standards has financial implications of considerable importance, especially when related to the complex insurance funding of hospitals in West Germany.

One significant hindrance, which applies especially to Europe, is the age of many of its institutions and the in-built traditions that are a consequence of this. A natural resistance to change, which is almost universal in organizations, is present, but reluctance to change may be soundly based: the latest trends may be ephemeral, may not produce worthwhile results, or may produce such results only at an unacceptably high cost. Both audit and staff appraisal are currently being subjected to critical scrutiny as to cost- effectiveness. Anyone who has become involved in the application of standards, is well aware of how costly it is in time and staff.

7. Intentions.

Our European colleagues are keen to develop to a high standard. Several mentioned the intention of setting up networks, or developing embryonic ones — Cyprus, Switzerland, Spain, Italy - thereby laying the foundations for improving existing conditions. Specifically, Greece has stated the aim to produce standards for the management and operation of libraries and the use of computers. Hungary was keen to introduce standards, and was eagerly awaiting this book, as was Bulgaria. Finland was embarking on a programme of library evaluation using an outside consultant, (the 1990 President of the UK Library Association, Maurice Line). Italy is aiming to promulgate the use of standard cataloguing rules and also create a directory of medical libraries and librarians. Directories too are essential tools in the early stages of standard preparation, as one is able to draw together a cohesive workforce with a common aim.

8. Quality Assurance.

Australia, Canada and the USA have published printed standards, on which quality assurance programmes are being created and these are described elsewhere in this book. However, because QA is an American term, many in Europe have not recognised the various activities in which they are already engaged as part of that process. A draft has been prepared by the King's Fund Centre on Accreditation of hospitals in the UK (King's Fund Centre 1989). The section on Libraries has been widely discussed. While being welcomed in the sense that any such proposed standards must in the end improve matters, a lot of the detail is inappropriate to the UK and automatically engenders suspicion and hostility. For example, it states that every employee must have a contract of employment as one of the standards. In the UK, by law, this is already the case. It reduces the validity of the document in question to state this, as it clearly has been lifted out of something that refers to another country's practice and indicates that the producer of the this "standard" was not in full possession of existing facts. This inevitably sows seeds of doubt as to the credibility of other parts of the document. The introduction to this document, however, clearly states that it is an early draft and invites comment and suggestion. As a result, many comments have been received and a useful dialogue has taken place.

Conclusions

As shown, Europe is very active in this field, albeit in a somewhat unco-ordinated way. Apart from the language problems mentioned in the intro-duction, Magalhães(1985) has made some penetrating observations which are so relevant and timely that no excuse is given for repeating them here. Europe is a country rich in diversity and subtlety. Part of that diversity is the two broad strands that are simultaneously complementary and antag-onistic: the "tectonic plates" of Anglo-Saxon attitudes and Latin culture. Libraries are essentially part of any organisation and, as such, are subject to an organisational ethos.

> "Organisation Development, which is a set of techniques and management strategies derived from Organisation Theory and from the practice of Management, was developed in an organ-isational culture which is traditionally open,liberal and with a preference for fairly loose organisational structures. Hence in Anglo-Saxon countries these techniques are welcome and they achieve positive results.... Many of the existing OD techniques are based on conditions of truth, trust, love and collaboration in the organisation. In Latin countries where the bureaucratic model prevails very strongly, these conditions are never found." (Magalhães, 1985)

As a member of the Council of the European Association of Health Infor-mation and Libraries I have had these cultural polarities confirmed. Quite serious misunderstandings developing due entirely to tone or different con-ventions. Standards can do no more than reflect the attitudes and aspirations of their creators. The inherent danger is that if they are transposed and laid on to another culture, there is unlikely to be a perfect fit. Trimming the pieces of a jigsaw puzzle to fit the gaps, produces a distorted picture which reflects uneasily the process whereby it was accomplished. This result is unlikely to gain the confidence of the people to whom the standards are meant to relate or who are meant to apply them. In these circumstances the standards promulgated will either be ignored or only lip service will be paid to them. This principle of appropriateness was discussed by Canisius (Magalhães 1985). Referring to the ultimately unsuccessful Unesco plan of 1974 for National Information Systems (NATIS), the following has direct relevance to our endeavours towards standards and QA.

a. before setting up any systems [read standards] all parties involved should be persuaded of their importance.

b. a flexible set of policies [standards] should be used, not a "policy".

c. production (ie results) rather than structures (i.e., organisational hierarchies) should be the target.

This echoes the "Körner" Committees in the UK which were set up in the late 1970s to examine the collection of NHS statistics. To put it bluntly, a great many NHS statistics were being collected which either revealed nothing, or were never used. The collection set has now been altered substantially and much more of what is being collected is being put to use. The evolution through standards to the attainment and maintenance of services of the highest quality is a worthwhile and practical goal. The fact that a "European" set of standards does not appear to be feasible given the impossibly wide variety of parameters with which it would have to cope, should not detract from the need to share and promote the highest quality possible.

We can use the skills and time others have spent and not go over the same ground endlessly, but adapt the relevant and add fresh ideas to areas unique to each one of us. We are engaged in doing our part in making the benefits of medical endeavour as widely available as possible.

Finally, there appear to be five vital facts which permeate the entire process of the creation of standards:

1. There is no such thing as a universal set of standards applicable throughout the world.

2. There are few absolutes and, unlike an exact science such as chemistry or electricity, much is based on the "best" example.

3. Standards need to be monitored, revised, upgraded, almost as a continuous process.

4. They must be accepted and respected by those called upon to use them.

5. When devising standards, reference can be made to work in other countries but great care must be taken not to transpose ideas and attitudes which are either culturally or economically unacceptable.

Acknowledgements

My thanks to colleagues in Belgium, Bulgaria, Cyprus, Denmark, Finland, France, Greece, Hungary, Irish Republic, Israel, Italy, Luxembourg, the Netherlands, Norway, Poland, Portugal, Spain, Switzerland, United Kingdom, Turkey, and Yugoslavia. Without their generous donation of time, interest and literature, this survey would not have been possible.

References

Adamic, S. and Gorec, S. (1988) Interlibrary lending in Yugoslav biomedical libraries in 1986. *Informatologia Yugoslavica,* **20**, 1–10.

Alberani, V. and Masciotta, O. (1986) *Biblioteche biomediche di Roma: Guida alle strutture organizzative e alle risorse bibliografiche.* Milano: Editrice Bibliografiche.

Brennan, P. W., Blackwelder, M. B., and Kirkali, M. (1987) Perspectives on medical school library services in Turkey. *Bulletin of the Medical Library Association,* **75**, 239–244.

Cavazza, L. (1990) Information service and bibliographical research in the libraries of Unita' Sanitarie Locali in Emilia-Romagna. A statistical survey. (In press.)

Council for Postgraduate Medical Education. (1981) *Desiderata for postgraduate medical centres.* CPME.

Egger, C. M. (1989) Die bibliotheksverkhaltnisse in den offentlichen Spitalern des Kantons Bern und der am klinischen Unterricht der Berner Fakultat beteiligten Spitaler Meducs 9 2 (3) 77–81

G.B. Department of Health (1989) *Accommodation for education and training Department of Health.* London: HMSO. (Health Building Note 42)

G.B. Department of Health. (1970) *Library services in hospitals.* Department of Health HM (70) 23 1970

King's Fund Centre. (1989) *Accreditation (UK) — Organisational audit. Quality Assurance programme project. Draft.* London: King's Fund Centre. (Report 89/52)

King's Fund Centre. (1990) Outline district audit programme. *British Medical Journal,* **300**, 382.

Library Association (1980) *Guidelines for library provision in the Health Service.* London: Library Association. (First published 1978)

Library Association (Annual) *Salary guide no 2. NHS library staff.* London: Library Association.

Magalhães, R. (1985) Change in library and information services: some thoughts on the Portugese scene. *Aslib Proceedings,* **37**, 181–194.

NHS/DHSS Health Services Information Steering Group. (1985) *Providing a district library service.* London: King's Fund Centre.

Ribes Cot, M. F., et al. (1990) The level of knowledge of medical documentation and the degree of usage of the library services on the part of medical residents, in: Stewart, D.W.C and Wright, D.J., eds. *Health information for all: a common goal. Proceedings of the Second European Conference of Medical Libraries, Bologna, Italy November 2–6 1988.* Munich: Saur. pp. 509–514.

Data collection for performance evaluation

Professor Tom Wilson
Head, Department of Information Studies,
University of Sheffield, U.K.

Service delivery as an experimental process

As other chapters in this book show, quality assurance is a multi-faceted set of performance measurement and assurance techniques. It might be thought of as nothing more than a fashionable buzz-word, like PPBS, MbO and zero-based budgeting. These topics once had their day in the literature but now little is written about them and it is difficult to know whether they have disappeared into the sediment of management techniques, or whether they survive in practice. Disappearance is almost guaranteed if we think of QA as simply a technique, but if it is viewed as an attitude of mind which governs the way we think about the management of library/information services, then it will survive in practice — so long as the measurement of performance is necessary.

In this respect, it is instructive to compare QA with action research. The stages of QA set out by Self and Gebhart (1980) can be compared almost directly with the stages of action research:

Quality Assurance

1. Select the subject for review and a sample population.

2. Develop measurable criteria.

3. Ratify the criteria.

49

4. Evaluate existing services using the criteria.

5. Identify problems.

6. Analyze problems.

7. Develop solutions.

8. Implement solutions.

9. Re-evaluate services.

Action Research

1. Identification of a problem area.

2. Selection of a specific problem in a way that implies a goal and a procedure for reaching it.

3. Record actions taken and accumulate evidence to determine the extent to which goal has been achieved.

4. Make inferences regarding relationships between actions and desired goal on the basis of the evidence.

5. Continuously retest the inferences through continued action. (Based on French and Bell, 1973)

The comparison of QA with action research is useful because no service should be implemented in the belief that it is going to remain unchanged. It is better to implement it in the spirit of experimentation and to see if it works, checking from time to time that it is still working as intended, that is, continuing to fulfill its function.

Central to the incorporation of QA into the librarian's philosophy of management is this notion of service delivery as an exploratory or experimental process. If we view every aspect of service as experimental, then how well the service satisfies its function will be a central question for management. The consequence is that it is necessary to collect data on the outcomes of service, as well as on the inputs to service. In other words, a broadly research approach will be necessary.

The role of data collection in QA

The term *data collection* is used here deliberately in place of the more common *research methods* because, from the point-of-view of the practicing librarian trying to find out what works and what doesn't, looking for ways to improve services, the word *research* has a number of irrelevant connotations. It brings to mind ideas of rigorous sampling, statistically valid data, generalization of results, and so on.

Of course, these are important concepts to consider when making claims for theories: but the librarian is looking for policy guidance rather than testing scientific theories. As a result, the rigorous requirements of research have to be loosened, partly because the practitioner lacks time to observe all the niceties of research methodology, partly because the information is needed within a limited time span, partly because the circumstances of the services and their user groups do not require them.

For example, the sample population in Self and Gebhart's terms, may be small enough to make nonsense of any idea of rigorous sampling. If a librarian is giving a specialized SDI service to five paediatricians, it would be silly to sample them. Hence, data collection rather than research.

Where, then, does data collection fit into performance evaluation? First, we have to know how much business we are doing in relation to any given service we offer, so we need to keep records, or, less time-consuming and just as accurate if done correctly, we need to sample activity at various times. Virtually any aspect of service is amenable to this kind of data collection, but the practice is much abused — data which are easy to collect are collected, but often not analyzed; circulation statistics are a case in point. On the other hand, data which are thought difficult to collect, for example, on the failure of clients to find what they are looking for in the collection, are often not collected at all.

Secondly, we need to know why the activity is at a given level and why clients are behaving the way they do in relation to any service. We need to know what they think about the services, how satisfactory they find them, what *they* mean by "satisfactory", and what criteria *they* would use to measure satisfaction or performance.

Thirdly, when changes are made to services, we need to discover what their effect is on levels of use. We can only do this by involving the clients in the process of change and by soliciting their views on the kinds of changes they would find useful.

Finally, when any change is implemented we need to know the consequences, either by comparing records of activity before the change with those collected afterwards, or by going back to clients and trying to discover whether they noticed the change and, if so, whether they respond positively or negatively to the changes made.

Methods of data collection

There are several good texts on research methods and their application to librarianship (for example, Busha and Harter, 1980; Martyn and Lancaster, 1981). There are hundreds more on research methods in general, and from either of these sets the librarian can learn much about data collection techniques. A chapter of this kind, therefore, is not the place to rehearse all of these methods, and theoretical ideas on the theoretically best way to do things may not be particularly useful. What the librarian wishing to evaluate performance needs to know is how to collect data in a way that will not be too time-consuming and that will be sufficient to produce data which will lead to sensible decisions.

Nor is it possible to review the various ways of collecting operational data. I have chosen, instead, to concentrate on survey methods, as these are the principal methods for collecting data from users — the ultimate judges of whether or not you are delivering quality services.

According to Self and Gebhart:

> "Four methods can be used to establish standards: (1) quantitative methods, (2) survey methods, (3) existing standards methods, and (4) qualitative methods."

This is an odd classification, and the authors go on to make an even odder statement:

> "Literature shows that the first three methods have not been useful in improving service."

Of course, no method of collecting data can, *of itself*, improve service: presumably the authors intended to say that information resulting from the first three methods had not proved useful in guiding decisions on how to improve services. But this is not true. There are certainly well-documented cases, at the University of Lancaster in the UK and at Purdue University in the USA, for example, where operational research (a quantitative method) most definitely led to improvement in services and there are other cases where surveys, particularly those using interviews, have led to the more detailed understanding of clients' needs and a consequent improvement in services.

At this point in their paper Self and Gebhart confuse data collection methods with finding answers to problems. Data collection results in data, analysis of which gives information which may or may not be useful in

decision-making, but which certainly cannot replace decision-making. And
what information is produced depends upon:

- how well the problem has been addressed,
- how well the objective of the study has been defined,
- how well the questions have been put to those involved in
  the evaluation, or
- how well any other data collection instrument, such as the
  recording format for an observational study, has been designed; and so on.

As with computers, so with surveys — garbage in, garbage out and,
similarly, if you do not know what you want to do with it (computer or
data) you might as well not bother with it in the first place.

I use a different classification of methods: all data are collected through
some form of observation, and within this major class, the investigator either
watches what happens, or she asks questions to seek *self-observations* from
the client. The questions usually ask someone to reflect upon what has
happened, or is happening, what is thought, what judgments are made,
what opinions are held, and so forth.

Observation

Observation is usually identified as a "qualitative" method; that is, one that
produces not data but some kind of account. The classic accounts are those
of the social anthropologist, the field-notes of his experiences in some strange
society, which can vary from a head-hunting tribe to a Welsh mining village.
In fact, observation can also produce quantitative data if that is what we
want.

For the librarian, observation is perhaps one of the most straight-forward
methods to use and, of course, we do it all the time, **but rarely bother
to record our observations**. When we give information to a client we
observe his/her behaviour: is s/he satisfied with the response? Is there
some uncertainty that suggests a problem in assimilating the information?
Is the "Thank you" genuine, or token, or ironic? It is a short step from
thinking about these aspects of service delivery to the design of a simple
data-recording format which can be used to identify problem areas and from
that point to the design of an interview schedule which can be used to follow
up with a wider range of clients than those observed.

Observation can be used whenever the client is in direct contact with some aspect of service and can be useful in gaining at least a preliminary idea of the quality of service. For example, is the catalogue used by those for whom it is intended? What is the behaviour of someone using the catalogue? Does any shelf search result from a catalogue search, or does the user record a citation? Do clients use the reference collection and, if so, which titles appear to be most used? Again, questions like this suggest themselves as elements of an observation check-list to be followed up later by other methods which involve asking questions directly of clients.

Librarians in different settings and different types of libraries have different opportunities to observe the behaviour of those they serve. The special librarian has the best opportunities because it is a relatively easy matter to walk around the organization with open eyes and ears. It is rather more difficult for the academic librarian to get into the workplace of the user and to see how information materials are being used, and even more difficult for the public librarian to do this, except perhaps in very limited cases. However, it is a fact that one learns more about why information is being sought and how it is used by being in contact with the client group than by remaining "at home" in the library. When I worked in an industrial research organization the Director said that I should spend one third of my time in the laboratories talking to people. "Otherwise," he said, "you won't know what's going on." He understood the value of observation, in its widest sense, for the information worker.

Anyone can do it because we all have the basic skill which we use every day of our lives: we just need to develop that skill and ask ourselves questions about the things we see. Take a stroll around the organization. Visit offices: how many items from the library are lying around? Are they being used? If so, ask about it: what is the client doing with the book or journal, how is it of use? If you have just sent out an information bulletin, where is it? Is it open on the desk, buried in the in-tray, or already in the waste-paper basket?

When doing tours like this (something which senior managers in industry are advised to do regularly) people tend to seize the moment and bring their information problems to you — if they know who you are. You can then discover how those information problems fit into the person's work, how important the problem is, what kind of information will be of use, and, indeed, as much as you care to ask about. Personal contact of this kind is a far better source of information on what you can do to improve quality of service than virtually any other form of data-gathering.

Every member of staff can observe and question and respond to needs in this way. A common response to this idea, however, is, "We don't have the time", to which there are two answers: first, you do not have to do it all the time — just now and again. Try it for an hour one week, do it again a few weeks later, wait a couple of months and do it again. Send out other members of staff to do it when you, the librarian, cannot — they might enjoy it and develop a new perception of their role in the organization. The second answer is that if you do not find time to do it, how do you know that the things you do find time for are worth doing? There is the further point that if you do not have time to watch what is going on you will not have a very good basis of understanding of the clients and their problems. This lack of understanding will make if more difficult for you to develop more structured methods of data collection.

Observation, then, is fundamental to our understanding of the situation in which we work, and fundamental to the process of developing methods of data collection which will provide more comprehensive data for management decisions. For reports on observational studies, see Wilson and Streatfield, 1981 and Streatfield, 1990.

Diaries

Diaries can also be considered an observation technique because in using a diary form we are asking the client to observe him/herself, and to report on those observations in some structured way. Usually, the structure is determined by the investigator, in this case the librarian. What kinds of observations are called for depends on what the librarian wants to know. It appeals as a method because the client has to do all the work — or so it seems. In fact, deciding what you want to know is probably the most difficult and time-consuming part of any investigation.

In the case of performance measurement the librarian wants to know what the client needs, whether he has difficulty in getting the material or the information, whether he is satisfied with what is obtained, among other things. The naive investigator might well think of trying to combine all of these points in a single diary form, but each needs to be the subject of separate investigation if clients are not to be overwhelmed by the task of completing the diary. If the burden of completion is too heavy the task will be rejected and no data will be obtained.

So, a simple diary study would involve asking the client to record all instances of needs for information of any kind on the diary form in a given

period (a week is usually the maximum period of time during which interest will be retained). The resulting form would have a simple four-column
design as in Figure 1. Each column heading replaces the questions in a
questionnaire. We are asking the client to respond to the questions:

- what is the date?
- what is the time?
- what problem is giving rise to a need for information? and,
- what information do you believe is necessary to answer the
  problem?

```
 ----------------------------------------------------------------
| Date |  Time  |    Problem    |    Needed Information    |
 ----------------------------------------------------------------
|      |        |      |        |      |        |        |      |
|      |        |      |        |      |        |        |      |
|      |        |      |        |      |        |        |      |
```

Figure 1: A diary format

"Time" is a useful category because analysis of the data may reveal something of the working day of people in the organization which may be relevant
to the design of services. For example, it is useful to know the pattern of
clients' working days, simply from the point-of-view of being able to make
contact when needed information is available. The problem statements will
reveal the range of concerns of clients of which the librarian may be unaware,
or where the client has been unaware that the librarian could help with a
given class of problems. Clearly, simple designs like this can be used to get
information relevant to all kinds of questions. Above all, the KISS principle
ought to be followed — "Keep it simple, stupid" — if clients have to read an
instruction manual on how to fill in the form they are not going to bother.

Earlier, I used the words "...for a limited period of time". The librarian
must remember that time is important to people and the shorter the period
of time over which you seek their cooperation in a diary study, the more
likely you are to get that cooperation. The kind of task outlined above
demands time of the client to complete the form, and requires that he should
remember to do so whenever appropriate instances of need arise. The time

taken to help you could otherwise be devoted to work, or to actually finding the needed information. It is better, therefore, to give the task to everyone for a day than to take a sample and ask each member of the sample to fill in the diary for a week. If the days are sampled over a working month, the data should reflect pretty accurately the pattern of work in the target group of clients.

Some years ago Dick Orr of the Institute for the Advancement of Medical Communication devised an ingenious method for encouraging people to respond to a very simple diary study. It involved the use of a "Random Alarm Mechanism" (RAM) which sounded a buzzer at random intervals during the day. Participants in the study were asked to tick a box on a response sheet, small enough to fit into the back of the RAM, asked what the user was doing when the buzzer sounded (Orr, 1970). Because of a carefully worked out time-sampling technique, the resulting data were valid and reliable, without undue pressure being put upon the survey participants. A similar technique was used in a study of reference library enquiries, using not a RAM (unavailable in the U.K.) but a cheap parking-meter timer (Wilson and Marsterson, 1973). The data obtained in that study were as accurate in identifying categories of enquiry as a previous study in which *every* enquiry was recorded by the library staff.

Asking questions

Questions are a normal part of any observation technique other than truly non-participant observation: after all, if you are unable to tell what is happening, it makes sense to ask. This point is made because it draws attention to the fact that the amount of structure we impose upon an investigation may vary. At one end of the spectrum is observation where we extract varying amounts of data from the events that go on around us, and where those events are not controlled by the researcher. At the other end is the highly structured questionnaire or interview schedule, which prompts the respondent to discuss *only* those matters which the researcher has decided are appropriate.

The amount of structure we impose upon an investigation, therefore, will determine the form, number and content of the questions we ask. Naturally, the amount of structure we impose is determined by what we want to achieve, what kind of data we intend to gather.

Although the term *questionnaire* is used to mean both instruments that are used in mail surveys and those used in interview surveys, it is useful to distinguish between the two by referring to the latter as *interview schedules.* This emphasizes the different characters of the two data collection activities. One instrument is used, and mainly completed, by an interviewer who is able to interpret questions to a degree and who is (or ought to be) adequately trained to use appropriate probes for further information. The other is completed by the respondent without any such assistance. This puts quite severe limitations on the kinds of questions that can be asked and demands that considerable attention be paid to removing ambiguity from the wording.

The literature on questionnaire design is extensive and more complex than can be dealt with here (for example, Hoinville et al., 1978; Oppenheim, 1970, and Payne, 1951). However, all agree on the key points of questionnaire design:

- Questions must be worded in such a way as to minimize the possibility of ambiguity.

- Questions must avoid jargon, except where the population to be studied is likely to use specialized jargon.

- The questions in an interview schedule must be easy for the interviewer to read — they must be written in *oral* language.

- A questionnaire should be composed of a logical sequence of questions, divided, where necessary, into a logical sequence of modules.

- Each module in a questionnaire should have a brief introduction to the content and aims of that module.

- Questions which solicit personal data should be in the final module of a questionnaire, *not* at the beginning.

- In a questionnaire where some questions act as "filter" (i.e. where the next question to be answered is determined by the answer to the filter question), the logical structure is best preserved by using arrows to the next question, rather than "Go to" instructions.

Interviewing

An interview is more than a conversation, although it shares some of the same characteristics: it involves two people, and there is interpersonal interaction, as well as verbal interaction. However, the interview is a directed conversation. The researcher has devised a set of questions, set these out in an interview schedule, and intends the "conversation" to follow the sequence of questions, and to provide information and data for research purposes, or, in the case of performance evaluation, for management purposes.

Interviewing has definite advantages over the use of mailed, self-completed questionnaires. It is possible to get more information (even to the same questions), and it is possible to prompt and probe to clarify the answers. It is also more expensive, of course, since it is necessary to spend time carrying out the interviews and, possibly, to buy that time. However, in terms of the quality of the information obtained, it may be worth the additional expense. The fundamental rule is that, if you know little about the area to be investigated, you must first carry out interviews and only use self-completed questionnaires when the problem area is more clearly defined and more properly understood.

There are numerous books on interviewing to guide the novice (a good starting point is Brenner et al., 1985), but, as with books on questionnaire design, there are some common rules to observe which provide a starting point:

- Always make appointments to interview. This is time consuming, but saves the waste of time involved in simply going looking for people. The exception is where you are interviewing in a public area, simply seeking clients who are prepared to be interviewed on the spot.

- When interviewing in offices, always try to carry out the interview without the presence of other people. If an office is open-plan, try to find an interview room. In public places, take the client aside to a quieter, traffic free spot.

- Make sure that you can see the interviewee's face. Don't sit so that his/her head is backed by a window. Non-verbal signs are often conveyed in facial movements.

- If you are using a tape-recorder, always ask for permission to do so.

- Explain the purpose of the interview, even if this has previously been set out in a letter.

- Ask the questions at a controlled, but not too slow, speed. Give proper emphasis to key words in the question.

- Never reveal any judgement of a response as good or bad, or typical or untypical. Never reveal surprise or unease at a response. You are looking for the interviewee's judgements and must supress your own.

- Record the answers you get verbatim, or as near to this as you can achieve.

- Probe for further information when you think more should have been said, but do so without *directing* the interviewee to a particular response.

- Read back the answer, especially when it is a fairly long one, and note any corrections made by the interviewee.

- Don't rush the interviewee into a response. If there is a period of silence - wait.

- Don't panic!

The mail survey

A mail survey, using a self-completed questionnaire, will be cheaper than interviewing and can be used if you know exactly how to ask the questions in ways that will be understood by respondents. The main problem is getting enough responses to be sure that you do not have a biased sample.

Many surveys appear to be satisfied with response rates well below 50%, and there are circumstances in which it may be difficult to achieve more than this. However, there is a well- established method of securing higher response rates, which is easy, if expensive, to implement. When you are carrying out a survey within a single organization, such as a hospital or a firm, the additional expense is minimal. The method was set out by Robin (1965):

- Before sending out the questionnaire, send out a "warning" letter, which tells the respondent that a questionnaire is on its way. *But do not give sufficient time for a response which says "I don't want the questionnaire".*

- Send out the questionnaire with a reply-paid envelope (where necessary) and a covering letter which repeats some of the information in the first letter.

- When the initial response tails off, send the first follow-up letter, with another covering letter that asks the respondent to use the original reply-paid envelope for the response.

- When the resultant surge of responses drops off, send the second follow-up letter, with another copy of the questionnaire and another reply-paid envelope.

- Repeat this a third time, if necessary, and if there is still time.

- Never give the impression that the follow-up letter will be the last to be sent out. Give the impression that this is the latest in a potentially infinite series.

Using this technique, very high response rates have been achieved, even in surveys of the general population. In any organizational study, it should be possible to achieve response rates well above 70%.

Coping with the data

Quantitative data

There is no space in a chapter such as this to delve into the mysteries of statistical analysis. Good guides to statistics are numerous, for example, Moroney, 1965 and Siegel and Castellan, 1988, but the best guide is a statistician. If you need advice, you may find that there is someone in your organization who is skilled in this area, or you may find that a local university or college offers a statistical advisory service.

Of course, there are micro-computer packages for statistical analysis, SPSS-PC+ being the best known, but you have to know what you are doing to get the best out of them. A golden rule, particularly in the relatively straightforward kind of data collection needed for management purposes, is to keep the analysis simple. Don't try to impress, simply report the data in a matter-of-fact way and give measures such as the mode and the mean, and the results of tests such as Chi-squared, only when they are actually justified.

Qualitative data

This is the *really* difficult part! Observation and interviewing give rise to textual information in the form of field notes and extended answers to questions. These cannot be analysed statistically, as they stand. Two strategies are available for coping with these kinds of data.

"Narrative accounts".

These are straightforward descriptive accounts of events, or of reported statements. This method was adopted in the Project INISS study of social workers and their managers (Wilson and Streatfield, 1981) in the observation
phase of the study, and those who had been observed found them both accurate and useful. The accounts were then combined into a fictionalized "week
in the life of" a social services department, as part of the final report to
the funding agency. The difficult part, of course, is the initial analysis of
the field notes to identify categories of behaviour, or whatever, under which
report can be made. The second strategy, outlined below, may be helpful
here.

Concept analysis or "topic cataloguing"

In this method, the aim is to take from the text, extracts and terms which
identify a particular kind of response or event. The work is time-consuming
and can be rather tedious — but the same can be said of much research!
The manual method is the easiest to explain and, unless you have all notes
or extended responses in a word-processor file, or unless you are using a
computer package such as *askSam* or *Ethnographer*, is the most likely to be
used.

Briefly, take a pack of 5 x 3 (or larger) cards and pick out quotations
which appear to be interesting, assigning each to a working category (or
categories) as you go along. After dealing with, say, three or four interview
schedules in this way, review the working categories and arrange the cards
under these categories in a sequence that has some meaning for you. For example, you may have asked respondents what they think of the usefulness of
a current-awareness bulletin and the responses may fall into two broad categories which you label for convenience, "Usefulness" and "Non-usefulness".
Group under the first head working categories such as "Time-saving", "Wide
scope", "Easy scanning", or whatever categories occur as you work through
the responses. Finally, review the categories, combine those that are closely
related and split those that seem to have useful conceptual subdivisions.
When this is done, writing the final report will seem like child's play!

If you do have a package like *askSam*, or indeed any other free-text
retrieval package, you can assign keywords to extracts and organize the whole
thing much more rapidly and effectively. *askSam's* hypertext capability is
useful for selecting quotations with common words, without requiring the

assignment of keywords, and in any free-text retrieval package you ought to be able to accomplish the same result by formulating search strategies.

Conclusion

I have tried to show that collecting performance data, especially data from the users of services, is a task which is well within the compass of the skilled librarian or information manager. To be sure, it is time-consuming, but so is the whole process of performance evaluation, and data-collection is an essential part of the process. If the task is well thought out and limited in scope to what can be achieved in the time available, and with the person-power available, then it is possible to get information from clients which can help to identify service strengths and weaknesses.

An earlier version of this paper was presented to a meeting of the Ontario Hospital Libraries Association in 1986.

References

Brenner, M., et al., eds. (1985) *The research interview: uses and approaches.* London: Academic Press.

Busha, C.H. and Harter, S.P. (1980) *Research methods in librarianship: techniques and interpretation.* New York: Academic Press.

French, W.L. and Bell, C.H. (1973) *Organization development.* Englewood Cliffs, N.J.: Prentice-Hall.

Hoinville, G., et al. (1978) *Survey research practice.* London: Heinemann.

Martyn, J. and Lancaster, F.W. (1981) *Investigative methods in library and information science: an introduction.* Arlington, VA.: Information Resources Press.

Moroney, M.J. (1965) *Facts from figures.* Harmondsworth, Middlesex: Penguin Books.

Oppenheim, A.N. (1970) *Questionnaire design and attitude measurement.* London: Heinemann.

Orr, R.H. (1970) The scientist as information processor: a conceptual model illustrated with data on variables related to library utilization, in:

Communication among scientists and engineers, edited by C.E. Nelson and D.K. Pollock. Lexington, MA.: Heath. pp.143–189.

Payne, S.L. (1951) *The art of asking questions.* Princeton, N. J.: Princeton University Press.

Robin, S.S. (1965) A procedure for securing returns to mail questionnaires. *Sociology and Social Research,* **50**, 24–36.

Self, P.C. and Gebhart, K.A. (1980) A quality assurance process in health sciences libraries. *Bulletin of the Medical Libraries Association,* **68**, 288–292.

Siegel, S. and Castellan, N.J. (1988) *Nonparametric statistics for the behavioral sciences.* New York: McGraw-Hill.

Streatfield, D.R. (1990) Observation and after, in: *Research methods in library and information studies,* edited by Margaret Slater. London: Library Association. pp.148–165.

Wilson, T.D. and Streatfield, D.R. (1981) Structured observation in the investigation of information needs. *Social Science Information Studies,* **1**, 173–184.

Wilson, T.D., et al. (1974) *Local library cooperation: final report on a project funded by the Department of Education and Science.* Sheffield: Postgraduate School of Librarianship and Information Science.

Performance indicators for the health care library: the macro dimension

John van Loo
Librarian, United Medical and Dental School of Guy's
and St. Thomas's Hospitals, London, U.K.

Introduction

Using quantitative performance measures to make judgements about the effectiveness and quality of services is not a new phenomenon in the health service. Florence Nightingale, for instance, used performance measures in the 1860s when she introduced a classification of "relieved/unrelieved/died" to evaluate the outcome of hospital care (Rosser, 1983).

Librarians are inveterate "counters", and there is a plethora of published work on performance measures, (see bibliographies by Reynolds, 1970 (184 references); Evans, 1972 (500 references); Ward, 1982 (220 references); Goodall, 1988 (59 references)). The National Health Service (NHS) library sector is not untypical of the international picture Goodall paints when she says:

> "...it would be wrong to suggest that no real progress has been
> made in the field of performance measurement but one cannot
> help feeling that the research has been of a circular nature and
> that although plenty has been written on the subject there is a
> surprising lack of originality in the writings. The research ap-
> pears to be collateral rather than cumulative; it is too often the
> case that old ideas are regurgitated with modifications rather
> than improvements." (Goodall, 1988)

Perhaps, more pertinently, it is the motivation of practising librarians
which should be criticised rather than the skills of their publishing colleagues,
as suggested by Cronin:

> "...it seems to us that the relative failure to utilize these tools (of
> performance measurement) has less to do with their dispersal in
> the primary literature than with the lack of practitioner interest
> in applying them to live situations." (Cronin, 1982)

Wessex and Oxford NHS Regions have published data (Robertson, 1978,
van Loo, 1988) and in 1988 the NHS Regional Librarians Group (RLG)
issued a Minimum Data Set for statistical workload collection for use by
NHS libraries, in an attempt to generate comparative data on a national
basis. The outcome of these initiatives is described later.

Some of the more useful, available performance data on health area libraries, which could provide comparative or trend data for library managers,
includes work on journal collection evaluation (Besson and Sherriff, 1986,
Fabrizio, 1985); a user survey (Brember and Leggate, 1985); document delivery work (Orr and Schless, 1972); book availability (Kolner and Welch,
1985); circulation and reference requests (Manthey and Brown, 1985); user
satisfaction (Dumais, 1986) and productivity measures (Phillips, 1990). The
greater number of publications on the development of hospital library standards and the evaluation of medical information retrieval systems is not part
of the remit of this paper.

This chapter, therefore, is an exhortation to develop and publish quantitative performance indicators in health care libraries as part of a general
commitment to improve the quality and responsiveness of library services. It
offers a rationale and guide for that purpose, and shares experience of work
undertaken at Regional and National levels.

The nature of performance indicators

Performance indicators can be used in various evaluation methods available to library managers, including peer review, audit, performance appraisal and external accreditation. They should not be seen as a simple method which provides solutions to questions of quality and value. The evaluation of library systems and services consists of judgements based on an aggregation of data grounded in three perspectives on the library:

- as a social mechanism (how users behave, interact and benefit);
- as a scientific process (how well indexing and information retrieval processes function); and
- as an economic-political system (accountability in allocating finite resources to meet infinite demand).

As Bawden (1990) persuasively argues and McElroy (1982) demonstrates, an holistic approach using a range of methodologies will pay dividends.

Quantitative performance indicators gain much of their meaning from the economic-political imperative and the logic of this model has been neatly demonstrated (Ford, 1989) by posing a series of questions, the answers to which are used to justify the library's funding:

- what is the library for?
- how should resources be allocated to help the library achieve its purpose?
- how well is the library achieving its purpose?
- how can we measure how well the library is achieving its purpose?
- what activities help the library achieve its purpose?
- how well is the library carrying out these activities?
- how can the performance of each activity be measured?

Bawden identifies a number of attributes of performance evaluation which give insights into the place of performance indicators and, of course, their limitations within the portfolio of performance measures (Bawden, 1990). These attributes can be represented on a series of continua:

- qualitative....................quantitative

- laboratory....................operational

- proof-oriented...............insight-oriented

- micro level....................macro level

- subjective....................objective

Performance indicators fall towards the right hand side of the scale of each of these attributes. The data are quantitative in measuring individual items; operational in measuring a real situation; insight-oriented in providing feedback rather than providing a conclusion; they have a macro-orientation in asking general questions about capability; and they are objective in providing data from which judgements can be made, which is not, and should not be, value-laden.

The Committee of Vice-Chancellors and Principals/University Grants Committee Working Party in their First Statement on Performance Indicators (CVCP, 1986) argued the case as follows:

> "Within the public domain attention has focussed on means of obtaining useful guidance in relation to the key issue of value for money and accountability. One mechanism for deriving such guidance is the development of performance indicators which are statements, usually quantified, on resources employed and achievements secured in areas relevant to the particular objectives of the enterprise. The emphasis is on performance as distinct from intention, and on indicators as signals or guides rather than absolute measures."

The thesis of this chapter is that performance indicators are a fundamental tool at the macro level within the economic-political system model, providing evidence for managerial benefit, rather than prescription for change. Within the national (UK) framework they are fundamental at this early stage of development of health care libraries, to provide comparative data, as a basis for "norms" to assist with the upgrading of underdeveloped services, and as a learning tool and precursor for more sophisticated systems.

Defining concepts

It is necessary to introduce and clarify certain paired concepts at this stage, in particular the concepts of outputs and outcomes, effectiveness and efficiency, quality and value, criteria and standards, each of which has a specific meaning for performance measures.

The performance of a library is multi-faceted, and as a system, will have the following components:

- **Inputs:** financial resources, expressed in monetary terms or what it buys (staff, stock, equipment).

- **Processes:** the organisation and use of resources, management structure, classification systems, policies and procedures, networking arrangements, and user education.

- **Outputs:** the "products" (or utilization) of the library — loans, inter-library loans, literature searches, enquiries, registered readers, library visits.

- **Outcomes:** the impact of the library on the organisation, time saved, improved decisions, more knowledgeable workforce, and better patient care.

When evaluating the performance of an organisation, this model helpfully differentiates outputs from outcomes and also shifts attention away from input measures, where there is a tendency to assume bigger is better, and where the importance of the input-output relationship is not made explicit.

Performance indicators can be applied to each of the components of the system. Inputs are often the easiest of the system components to measure and much of the early published work on performance measures has been criticised because it concentrated on financial and resource inputs unrelated to library objectives (Knightly, 1979). Process relates to the activities required to translate inputs into outputs, and indicators measure recall and precision of retrieval systems, document delivery times, or, more commonly, the efficiency or cost-efficiency of procedures — inter-library loans, accessions, recruitment practices or automated circulation control systems. Outputs are a means to satisfying an end-product — the outcome. Measuring the performance of outputs (the use of the service) will be very different from measuring the performance of outcomes (the benefits of the service) and should not be confused.

Output and outcome relate to the objectives of the organisation and, therefore, its effectiveness. This must be differentiated from efficiency which is inward-looking (and usually a process measurement) and can be measured without reference to effectiveness. The book selection procedure can be efficient in time and cost, but if the appropiate stock is not being purchased the service is not contributing to the aims of the library. Effectiveness, therefore, relates directly to the achievement of objectives and cannot be considered outside a framework of predetermined performance targets or action plans.

A necessary insight into library performance assessment relates to the two components, quality and value, of what Orr calls "goodness" in one of the seminal works on performance measures (Orr, 1973). Quality relates to "the capability (of the library) for meeting the user needs it is intended to serve", and value relates to "the beneficial effects accruing from its use".

It is useful to keep this differentiation between quality and value in mind. Value (or benefit) is equivalent to outcome in the systems model and there is much debate on the practicality and feasibilty of measuring outcome (Blagden, 1980 gives an indication of the problems). The performance outcome of a health care library in organizational terms should reflect the objectives of the parent organization, i.e., to make a contribution to better patient care or to the improved health of the community, with sub-objectives of contributing to the educational/knowledge levels of health care staff, research results or management decision making. To effectively measure and demonstrate the causal relationship between libraries and these outcomes, if not impossible, would require resources and skills beyond our capacity. Is it the role of the librarian to ensure that information obtained from the library is used appropriately by the practitioner or manager? Potentially useful research in health care libraries in this area by applying the concepts of value added services and disbenefit of lack of information, in an attempt to put a monetary value on library information, should be noted (King, 1987, Banks, 1989).

The quality component of library performance can be measured more easily, as it relates to outputs, or to surrogate outcomes such as user satisfaction. Further useful analysis of the nature of quality is made by Maxwell (1984), who identifies six dimensions of quality in health care, each of which can be given a library performance context:

- access to services: use of services, hours open, network facilities;

- relevance to needs: differentiation of service provision between students, clinicians, managers;

- effectiveness for individuals: accuracy and timeliness of enquiries answered;

- equity: balance of resources between user groups;

- social acceptability: study environment, interpersonal skills of staff;

- efficiency: workload and unit cost comparisons.

The assessment of any of these aspects of the library system should operate within a planning process. Any general objectives (mission statements) need to be translated into specific elements which can be defined and measured. This involves establishing the objective, framing an action plan, implementing the programme , measuring the outcome, evaluating the outcome and redefining the objectives. Within this framework, criteria (the units which are measured), monitoring procedure (the data collection methodology) and standards (the target to be reached) will be set. For example, the objective may be to raise the profile of the library with Unit Managers. The criteria could be the librarian speaking at unit meetings and library use by unit managers; monitoring would be self-checking at meetings and a log of enquiries/loans at the library counter; and the standards might be to speak at 100% of meetings and to increase managers' enquiries by 10% within a six month period.

Standards can be used either as a minimum level or as a target to be achieved, and must therefore be used with great care. Difficulties in the use of standards include the speed with which they become out-dated, inflexibility in adapting to local circumstances, their orientation to input processes and emphasis on value-laden statements (bigger/more is better!) The real issue, in fact, is not one of defining the performance measure nor of data collection, but of applying the planning process.

"The problem of library measurement is not one of finding the right indicator to measure the library's success at meeting demand, but one of deciding which of the needs the library will aim to service and then of measuring what happens when the attempt to meet the chosen need is made." (Allred, 1979)

Context and use of performance indicators

Performance indicators are just one of several tools to evaluate services and improve their quality. Although there has been research into identifying a single, global measure for assessing services (for example, the derived value ratio (Wills and Oldman, 1977), book availability (Revill, 1987) and document exposure (Hamburg, 1972)), and although it has been argued that a single output measure is valuable for political purposes (van Loo, 1989), it is essential that a range of performance indicators be established which reflect different library demands and the interdependence of processes.

A useful checklist for devising performance measures is provided by Revill. He suggests librarians should concentrate on aspects of the service which:

- are time consuming
- need a great deal of space
- cost a lot of money
- affect a lot of users
- are directly related to library objectives
- are definable and easily described
- can be collected relatively easily
- are strongly affected by constraints over which the library staff have some control. (Revill, 1989)

A number of issues need to be faced when introducing a comprehensive system of performance indicators. They relate to their collection, analysis and publication.

Collection: The primary decision is concerned with what is to be collected. This should be the outcome of discussions on the objectives and sub-objectives of the service. There is considerable effort in data collection and the senior managers who analyse and present the data, first-line managers who maintain the system and clerical staff who collect the data must all understand and "own" the objectives before they can be expected to expend effort on an "administrative" task. The number of data elements to be collected, how specific they should be and the effort required to collect the data are also critical decisions. For instance, there are 180 NHS Health Service Indicators for the hospital sector alone; the Committee of

Vice-Chancellors and Principals have devised 30 for the University sector; and the NHS Training Authority have produced six indicators for training performance. The depth of detail is dependent on the need for information and the requirement for ongoing or ad hoc data collection. Automated systems will reduce the time spent on data collection and also help analysis. The management information spin-off from automation should be a major factor in its design and specification. Finally, the definition of each data element is fundamental. Each one must be totally unambiguous: for example, should a renewal of a book be counted as an additional loan? Should user groups be counted as full-time eqivalent numbers or by head count?

Analysis: Performance indicators can be used to show achievement of specific objectives or as one of a porfolio of tools to assess the general capability of services. Drawing meaningful conclusions is dependent on the selection of the right criteria, an understanding of the local situation, and the analytical skills of the manager. Thought should be given to presentation (graphs, charts, ratios), links with other evaluation methods and the speed of making the data available.

Publication: The political dimension of performance indicators must also be addressed. Who are the figures for? DHA managers, non-librarian library managers, library staff, and other librarians in the NHS will all have different perceptions, knowledge and values about the library service, and may therefore read different agendas into the data. Other important issues concern questions about who should have access to the raw data for analysis, is the analysis open to argument and debate and if there is feedback, is there a cycle of comment to allow amendment to the following year's collection?

An important and newly apparent issue is the ethical dimension of performance indicators. No information system is value-free and the choices which are made in collection, analysis and publication will affect the utility and capacity of the indicators. Clarity and relevance of objectives are critical to the choices of what is to be collected, who will analyse the data and how it will be disseminated.

These choices are particularly relevant at a time of major NHS structural changes which are being manifested through demands for value for money, financial accountablity, new contractual relationships and individual performance review. As professional librarians, we need to take the lead in specifying what a quality service consists of, how this can be measured and what standards should be set. Accountability, quality and performance indicators are thus inseparable within a professional framework, and place performance indicators securely at the core of managerial practice.

Performance indicators are one of the practical responses to the problem of translating the concepts of accountability, quality, effectiveness and
efficiency into specific action. They are of use as a means to an end but
therefore only gain meaning when acted upon — in other words, when they
are part of the planning process. An excellent practical guide from the nurse
education field, which emphasises these principles, has been produced by the
English National Board for Nursing and Midwifery (Balogh, 1989). It gives
worked examples of performance indicators, and suggests workshop activities
and discussion topics for further group learning.

Performance indicators in the Oxford Region Library and Information Service

The Oxford NHS Region comprises the administrative counties of Oxfordshire, Berkshire, Buckinghamshire and Northamptonshire and is divided into
eight District Health Authorities (DHA). It is one of the larger geographical
regions but the second smallest in population terms (2.5 million). Library
services, which serve the professional, managerial, research, support worker
and educational staff, are structured into seven "District Library Services"
plus the libraries in Oxfordshire (the teaching hospital District). Libraries
are co-ordinated at the Regional level by the Librarian/Co-ordinator, a joint
NHS/Oxford University appointment. In total there are 35 libraries with an
establishment of 65 staff (48.8 whole-time equivalent) and an expenditure of
c.£750,000 per annum.

A minimum data set of 19 workload activity measures has been collected by each library in the Oxford Region Library and Information Service
(ORLIS) since 1981-82, covering loans, inter- library loans and photocopies,
photocopies made by staff, online searches and stock accessions. An abridged
form of this data for the last four years for the whole network is presented in
Table 1, and demonstrates increasing workload activity, primarily in inter-
library photocopy activity (+29%), material obtained from within the Region (+28%) and book loans (+20%). The value of this has been to provide
a general overview of trends, to monitor use of the service, to assess the
ability of the network to be self-sufficient, to compare library services in the
network and to identify major differences from the norm. They are used
annually with the RHA (and their treasurers) to demonstrate the value and
scale of the activity in libraries, as evidence for increased resources and to
counter arguments for "cost improvements" by demonstrating the reduced

unit costs of library transactions. The figures are crude and require further breakdown and analysis, but they are the building blocks of more sophisticated performance evaluation in the form of ratios.

Function	1989-90	1988-89	1987-88	1986-87
Loans	91,502	82,327	74,898	76,057
Inter-library loans	4,863	4,936	4,776	4,963
Photocopies made	60,869	47,880	50,211	45,642
Photocopies rec'd	29,918	27,728	25,327	23,160
Accessions	11,544	10,473	8,982	8,934
Online searches	4,119	4,858	3,740	4,062
ORLIS ILLs: Books	1,875	1,545	1,884	1,407
ORLIS ILLs: PCs	14,549	13,039	12,476	11,377

Table 1: Workload statistics

Since 1984-85 resource measures have also been collected: number of library staff, book stock, journal titles, staff and non-staff expenditure, user population (all staff employed by a DHA) and NHS District expenditure.

These data elements are valuable because they provide the denominator for ratios which provide meaningful comparative information for libraries and Districts which vary in size. As an example, Table 2 gives nine of the ratios collected in 1989-90 derived from the data provided in Table 3, for the seven District Library Services. Thus, District A with a NHS staff population of 8580 and library expenditure of £112,400 can be compared with District E with a user population of 3120 and expenditure of £43,500. The average for the seven non-teaching Districts is also provided.

The nine ratios provide excellent analytical data for evaluations of the performance of the library services in the Oxford Region, relating inputs (income, stock, staff) to outputs (transactions). Library transactions are taken as the main indicator of output, and include all loans (to other libraries and to readers), material borrowed from other libraries and photocopies made by staff. Financial indicators (Table 2. Nos. 1, 2, and 6) express library expenditure as a percentage of the total DHA expenditure, library expenditure per user population head and staff expenditure as a percentage of total expenditure. Resource indicators (Table 2. Nos. 5, 7, and 8) provide valuable comparative intelligence on staffing and stock levels. A simple measure of activity within the library can be gauged by the workload ratios (Table 2. Nos. 3, and 4) which indicate the "busyness" of the library in terms of staff activity and impact within the user population.

	Districts							
Ratios	A	B	C	D	E	F	G	Ave.
1. Lib Exp as % Dist Exp	0.119	0.098	0.120	0.106	0.137	0.156	0.092	0.119
2. Per Cap Exp £	13.10	13.12	11.89	12.47	13.95	17.13	9.13	12.97
3. Trans Per Lib Staff	3603	3989	4266	7386	4639	3360	3855	4443
4. Trans Per NHS Staff	2.7	3.1	3.1	4.8	4.1	3.3	1.8	3.3
5. NHS Staff per Lib Staff	1320	1300	1360	1520	1130	1030	2200	1410
6. % Expend Lib Staff	60%	56%	67%	55%	63%	56%	51%	58%
7. Books Per NHS Staff	2.5	1.7	1.6	2.1	1.8	2.8	1.3	1.9
8. NHS Staff per Jnl.	20	20	27	17	24	22	25	22
9. ORLIS ILLs as % Total	39%	56%	51%	44%	62%	52%	69%	53%

Table 2: ORLIS performance ratios 1989–90

From the data presented a number of conclusions can be drawn — District G is significantly under-resourced and there are wide differentials between library services in levels of stock and workload. This raises questions for local management such as why some libraries are more active than others, why some libraries undertake more inter-library loans, how policies affect transaction patterns, but more especially what other indicators might reflect the impact of library services.

Referring back to the section on the nature of performance indicators and Bawden's attributes you will see that these data are primarily insight-oriented at the macro level. What is not available are data on the standard of stock, the skills of the librarian, the political strength of the library or the accuracy of any information provided.

In practical terms, although there seems to be a steady increase in resources, the allocation of additional funds has been patchy, and it is difficult

Districts							
Data	A	B	C	D	E	F	G
Library Expend £	112,400	71,600	50,200	56,400	43,500	113,200	41,700
Library Staff Exp £	67,600	40,000	33,700	30,900	27,500	63,400	21,200
District Expend £mil	94.573	73.034	41.908	53.284	31.708	72.699	45.211
NHS Users (Heads)	8580	5460	4230	4530	3120	6600	4570
Total Transactions	23,562	16,755	13,267	21,938	12,803	21,536	8,019
Book/Ph'cops ILLs	4192	3252	1741	2985	2498	3140	1517
BL Loans/Ph'cops	1398	909	591	956	826	1032	232
ORLIS Loans/Ph'cops	1651	1818	896	1326	1538	1639	1043
Library Staff (FTE)	6.54	4.21	3.11	2.97	2.76	6.41	2.08
Book Stock	21,560	9,290	6,610	9,500	5,670	18,750	6,100
Journal Titles	431	278	154	261	128	304	180

Table 3: ORLIS performance data 1989–90

to ascribe any funding increase to evidence derived from performance indicators directly, rather than the "political" way they have been used. In the changing management climate of the current NHS, with emphasis on cash limits, contracts, income generation and the internal market, proactive rather than reactive tools will be required. This may involve writing a specification and contract for library services, similar to that undertaken for paramedical services (Haywood, 1990) which includes:

- organizational goals and objectives
- service objectives
- national and regional policy guidance
- population to be served
- quality standards
- monitoring procedures
- resource needs/costs

NHS Regional Librarians Group

In 1986, following a request from the Library and Information Services Council (England) for activity and resource data from NHS libraries to sit alongside data from the University, Polytechnic and Public Library sectors in their Annual Report, the RLG agreed that a national minimum data set should be established and that all NHS and medical school libraries should be asked to complete this. The objectives for the collection of these data were:

- to provide data on the size of the market and scale of activity in NHS libraries for the RLG to use in their discussions and negotiations with other national bodies,

- to provide comparative data between Regions on staffing norms, regional ILLs, levels of stock etc, for use by individual Regional Librarians.

The retrospective collection of workload statistics for 1987-88 was requested and 341 library services made returns. This meant a return from at least one library in 81% of Districts/Boards in the UK. As expected, there were blank returns for some data elements and, therefore, the totals for each activity could only provide a minimum picture. For 1988-89 the returns increased to 419 library services, covering 87% of Districts/Boards, with the totals for each activity providing more reliable figures.

Analysis of these data is best achieved by translation into ratios for comparative purposes. Table 4 gives three ratios for NHS libraries in the 14 English Regions. It must be emphasised that these data are from an incomplete survey of libraries, some Regions making 100% responses, others 70%. In particular, for ratios 1 and 2 (where the denominator (NHS staff employed) is accurate for each Region, but where the numerator's accuracy is variable), any comparison must be made with knowledge of the local circumstances.

1. NHS library staff (full-time equivalent) per total NHS staff employed (DHSS, 1989: Table 3.2). A measure of the level of staff resources in each Region.

2. Transactions (loans, ILL's, photocopies) per NHS staff employed. A measure of the impact/visibility of the library service in the Region.

3. Inter-library loans from within the Region as a % of total ILL's, (includes ILLs from university medical school libraries). A measure of the

self-sufficiency of the Region in resource sharing and satisfying requests from its own libraries.

The following additional ratios are also available:

- **Inputs:** qualified library staff per NHS staff employed, bookstock/ journal titles per NHS staff employed.

- **Process:** transactions per library staff, BL ILLs as % of total ILLs.

- **Output:** loans, ILLs, online searches per NHS staff employed.

Ratio	1	2	3	Ratio	1	2	3
Region A	1620	1.91	37%	Region H	1114	3.00	38%
Region B	2134	2.33	24%*	Region I	1020	4.21	58%
Region C	1957	2.08	22%	Region J	1107	3.72	45%
Region D	1772	2.25	45%	Region K	1284	3.17	29%*
Region E	2936	1.13	27%	Region L	1509	3.09	54%
Region F	2116	1.49	54%	Region M	2197	1.07	19%
Region G	951	3.66	56%	Region N	1937	2.34	46%*

* Excludes university medical school ILL data

Table 4: Regional Performance Ratios 1988-89

More sophisticated statistical analysis can be undertaken to look at relationships between some of these results. For instance there is a positive correlation between number of library staff and total transactions undertaken, and also a positive correlation between number of journal titles taken and number of inter-library loans. Thus the more resources one provides (staff or journals) the greater the demand for services. Does this reflect the ability of the library to create demand or the provision of a more personal service to a wider client group?

Despite the useful insights of these data, the 87% response is discouraging (LISC for instance do not feel it is sufficiently comprehensive to include it in their Annual Report). A 1985 census of library staff (NHS Regional Librarians Group, 1987) identified 1023 libraries serving NHS staff. Bearing in mind that many of the small libraries will have been amalgamated and some returns will have been made on a District basis, 419 returns cannot be termed comprehensive. In fact only six out of the seventeen UK Regions were able to provide a 100% response from Districts/Boards in their Regions. Many library staff are apparently unconvinced that this type of performance data is relevant and useful, at least at the national level.

It is suggested that the reasons for this incomplete return on a national basis are related to:

1. Librarians being wary of giving performance data to a national body (although requested through Regional networks) where it may be interpreted without knowledge of the local context.

2. Librarians feeling personally threatened by the collection of performance data as this is related to accountability and value for money.

3. Librarians, not collecting any (or little) workload data and surviving without them, are not motivated or encouraged (by local management) to start.

4. Librarians having their own, but different workload measures, are reluctant to change practices.

5. Librarians holding the view that performance indicators are irrelevant, difficult to use and do not measure the qualitative nature of the service.

6. Librarians concerned that performance indicators lead to league tables that discriminate against those above the norm, and that the norm is used as the standard.

7. The effort is not worthwhile as the changes suggested cannot be implemented.

The lessons to be learnt from the RLG exercise are that the local libraries must "own" the collection of the data — any national minimum data-set must match local requirements. The local library must have identified the need to collect and analyse those data elements. Communication must be two-way, from the RLG regarding the objectives for their collection and the local benefits that will accrue, and from the collectors regarding problems in definitions or ambiguities. Finally results should be published and cascaded to all involved, so that the results of librarians' efforts can be seen and debated.

Conclusion

In conclusion, much further persuasion is required if performance indicators are to be adopted on a national scale within the health care sector. Three factors will help this to be achieved.

First, presentation of data (at local, regional and national level) should be improved so that all users (librarians, library committees, funders) find the information more meaningful and easier to assimilate. Second, training in the value, processes and analysis of data collection must be undertaken at a national level, and a recognition both of the skills and the time required for this task should be given. Third, further research must be undertaken into measures of the outcome of the provision of library services.

John van Loo was formerly Regional Services Librarian, Oxford Region Library and Information Service.

References

Allred, J. (1979) *The measurement of library services: an appraisal of curent possibilities and practices.* Bradford: MCB Publications.

Balogh, R., Beattie, A. and Beckerleg, S. (1989) *Figuring out performance: a guide to assessing performance and quality in nursing and midwifery training institutions.* London: ENB.

Banks, R. (1989) Measuring the impact of a hospital library in terms of value added processes. *Bibliotheca Medica Canadiana,* **10**, 184–190.

Bawden, D. (1990) *User oriented evaluation of information systems and services.* Aldershot: Gower.

Besson, A. and Sherriff, I. (1986) Journal collection evaluation at the Medical College of St. Bartholomew's Hospital. *British Journal of Academic Librarianship,* **1**, 132–43.

Blagden, J. (1980) *Do we really need libraries?* London: Bingley.

Brember, V. and Leggate, P. (1985) Linking a medical user survey to management for library effectiveness — 1: The user survey. *Journal of Documentation,* **41**, 1–14.

Committee of Vice-Chancellors and Principals. (1986) *Performance indicators in Universities: a first statement by a Joint CVCP/UGC Working*

Party. London: CVCP.

Cronin, B. (1982) Performance measurement and information management. *Aslib Proceedings,* **34**, 227–36.

Department of Health and Social Security (1989) *Health and personal social service statistics, 1989.* London: DHSS.

Dumais, M. (1986) Evaluation of the effectiveness of a small library. *Documentation et Bibliothèques,* **32**, 51–52.

Evans, E., Borko, H. and Ferguson, P. (1972) Review of criteria used to measure library effectiveness. *Bulletin of the Medical Library Association,* **60**, 102–110.

Fabrizio, N.A. (1985) Journal evaluation in a health sciences library. *Serials Review,* **11**, 55–57.

Ford, G. (1989) Performance measurement: principles and practice. *IFLA Journal,* **15**, 13–17.

Goodall, D.L. (1988) Performance measurement: a historical perspective. *Journal of Librarianship,* **20**, 128–145.

Hamburg, M., Ramist, L.E. and Bommer, R. W. (1972) Library objectives and performance measures and their use in decision making. *Library Quarterly,* **42**, 107–128.

Haywood, S.C. (1990) *Professions allied to medicine: contracts for services.* Birmingham: University of Birmingham, Health Services Management Centre.

King, D.N. (1987) The contribution of hospital library information services to clinical care: a study in eight hospitals. *Bulletin of the Medical Library Association,* **75**, 291–301.

Knightly, J.J. (1979) Overcoming the criterion problem in the evaluation of library performance. *Special Libraries,* **70**, 173–178.

Kolner, S.J. and Welch, E.C. (1985) The book availability study as an objective measure of performance in a health sciences library. *Bulletin of the Medical Library Association,* **73**, 121–131.

McElroy, A.R. (1982) Library – Information service evaluation: a case history from pharmaceutical R and D. *Aslib Proceedings,* **34**, 249–265.

Manthey, T. and Brown, J.O. (1985) Evaluating a special library using public library output measures. *Special Libraries,* **76**, 282–289.

Maxwell, R. (1984) Quality assessment in health. *British Medical Journal,* **288**, 1470–72.

NHS Regional Librarians Group. (1987) *Census of staff providing library services to NHS personnel: December 1985.* Guildford: NHS RLG.

Orr, R.H. (1973) Measuring the goodness of library services: a general framework for considering quantitative measures. *Journal of Documentation,* **29**, 315–332.

Orr, R.H. and Schless, A.P. (1972) Document delivery capabilities of major biomedical libraries in 1968. Results of a national survey employing standardised tests. *Bulletin of the Medical Library Association,* **60**, 382–422.

Phillips, S.A. (1990) Productivity measurement in hospital libraries: a case report. *Bulletin of the Medical Library Association,* **78**, 146–153.

Revill, D. H. (1987) "Availability" as a performance measure for academic libraries. *Journal of Librarianship,* **19**, 14–30.

Revill, D. (1989) What should we evaluate, and how? People, materials, services, in: Brewer, J.G., ed. *Evaluating library and learning resource services — papers presented at the CoFHE Annual Study Conference 1988.* London: Library Association, Colleges of Further and Higher Education Group.

Reynolds, R.A. (1970) *A selective bibliography on measurement in library and information services.* London: Aslib.

Robertson, E. M. (1978) Measurement and monitoring, in: Tabor, R.B., ed. *Libraries for health: the Wessex experience.* Southampton: Wessex Regional Library and Information Service.

Rosser, R.M. (1983) A history of the development of health indicators, in: Teeling-Smith, G., ed. *Measuring the social benefits of medicine.* London: Office of Health Economics.

van Loo, J. (1988) Performance indicators in the Oxford Region Library and Information service: first steps. *Health Libraries Review,* **5**, 221–225.

van Loo, J. (1989) Performance measurement: can you manage without it? Library and Information Research Group Conference Report. November 1988. *Health Libraries Review,* **6**, 95–96.

Ward, P.L., ed. (1982) *Performance measures: a bibliography.* Loughborough: Loughborough University of Technology, Centre for Library and Information Management. (CLAIM Report No. 13)

Wills, G. and Oldman, C. (1977) *The beneficial library: a methodological investigation to identify ways of measuring the benefits provided by libraries.* Cranfield: Cranfield School of Management. (BL R & D Report No. 5389)

Database search services: a quality assurance approach

Joanne G. Marshall
Faculty of Library and Information Science,
University of Toronto, Ontario, Canada

Introduction

The purpose of this chapter is to apply the principles of evaluation and quality assurance (QA) to an important component of library and information services, namely the provision of electronic database searches. Database services are first discussed in the context of library reference services. Various approaches that have been taken to the evaluation of reference and database search services are reviewed and the differences between these approaches and QA are noted. The application of QA principles to database search services to date has been very limited but a recent report by Humphries and Naisawald (forthcoming) is described as a model.

The notion of producing a "quality product" through careful monitoring and control of manufacturing processes has been a key operating principle in industry for many years. The application of this approach to human services, as opposed to assembly-line production, obviously presents a new and different set of challenges. Evaluation techniques such as QA, utilization review and peer review have been used in the health field for some years to monitor and upgrade services and to assist in managerial decision-making. While health has not been the only service sector to adopt these approaches, health-care organizations have developed one of the most elaborate QA systems. Librarians within these organizations have been among the first to apply these principles to the provision of library services. Since there is a growing concern about evaluating library and information services in general, approaches such as QA deserve attention not only from health sciences librarians, but also from librarians and information specialists in other settings.

Other chapters in this book provide a fuller description of the history and development of QA and the related field of performance measurement; nevertheless it is useful to review the main principles of QA as a basis for a discussion of database search services. As Eagleton (1988) points out, the concept of QA in health-care in North America emerged between the mid-seventies and mid-eighties as an elaboration of existing standards for hospital accreditation. Whereas earlier standards emphasized the type and quantity of patient care services to be provided in institutional settings, the QA approach enlarged the scope of the standards to include "quality of care". The QA process entailed establishing hospital-wide quality standards, initiating procedures to ensure that these standards were achieved and, if they were not, having additional procedures in place for taking remedial action. Among the principles of QA programmes were: that they should be administered by the hospital staff members themselves; that they should be ongoing and continuous; and that they should be tailored to the needs and structure of the particular institution.

QA, which strives to assure the adequacy of both the quantity and quality of services has become a laudable and even necessary goal for organizations that provide critical human services such as hospitals and other health-care facilities. But the time and effort required to implement these systems has also proved to be substantial. Many health-care institutions have QA directors who work full time on the development and maintenance of QA programmes with the various clinical department heads. Librarians in these institutions also work with the QA director to develop library service QA standards, monitoring procedures and plans for remedial action.

Database search services

The phrase "database search services" is used in this chapter to describe the variety of electronic information services that can be provided by libraries today. Database search services originated in the late sixties and early seventies when producers of major bibliographic indexing and abstracting services discovered the computer. Computers are amazingly adept at storing and sorting large amounts of information in a variety of ways which is exactly what producers of indexing tools require for the preparation of their printed publications. Once these data are in machine-readable form, the possibility of searching them electronically also exists, assuming that the user can connect to the host computer where the data are stored. These early databases were primarily bibliographic, supplying information such as the author, title and source of the original documents. Today there is an increasing trend towards the production of full-text databases that contain the documents themselves.

Bibliographic and full-text databases have always required large amounts of electronic storage, more than the typical microcomputer has available. Until recently, this meant that the databases had to be stored centrally on a host computer with data terminals or microcomputers used to access them. Since the searcher's equipment was connected to the host computer via a telephone line, the term "online" was used to describe the connection between the user and the search system. Offline searches were also available in which the searcher would input the search request "online" and the host computer would process the search "offline", usually during off-peak hours when fewer users were connected to the system. The offline search results would be mailed the next day. Online search services developed primarily as intermediary services in which a librarian or information specialist conducted the search for the user.

In the mid-eighties, a new trend emerged toward end-user online searching, or direct database searching by the person who needs the information. This development was supported by other trends toward the increasing use of microcomputers in work settings and the recognition of information as an important organizational resource. Another significant development affecting database search services has been the increasing availability of CD-ROM(Compact Disc - Read Only Memory) products. CD-ROMis a new mass storage medium that allows on site storage of large databases. CD-ROMis a microcomputer peripheral, i.e., a CD-ROMdrive is connected to a microcomputer which acts as the access device for the CD-ROM. In addition, CD-ROM does not require a telephone connection as does database searching on a remote host computer.

While end-user online searching was a trend with the potential to take users away from the library because they could perform searches on their own equipment in their own offices, CD-ROM may well bring these same users back into the library. This is because the cost of subscriptions to CD-ROM databases (often $1,000 US annually or more, depending on the database) makes purchase by individual end-users unlikely at present. CD-ROM is, of

course, only one form of mass local electronic storage and there may soon
be others that prove to be superior in one way or another.

A final change that is affecting the original approach to online search
service is the trend towards the mounting of large databases locally by academic libraries and other libraries with a substantial user base. Many large
libraries now have online public access catalogues (OPAC'S) that provide access to the book and serial titles held in the library. Once an OPAC is in place,
it is possible to mount other commercially-available databases in the same
electronic environment so that a library user could first search the library's
catalogue for books and then move on to search the appropriate database
for the journal literature, such as ERIC, MEDLINE, INSPEC OR PSYCINFO.

In this dramatically changing world of database searching — from intermediary to end user — from remote host computer to local access — from
bibliographic to full text — how can database search services in libraries
be defined? Many libraries still refer to their database search services as
online services; however the literature is full of discussions on the impact of
CD-ROMand end-user searching on mediated library search services. Clearly,
the nature and type of electronic access provided by libraries is changing
rapidly. Mediated online search services are now only one part of a range of
services that librarians provide. A potential list of services is shown below:

1. Automated search service

2. Provision and maintenance of end-user workstations (online
   or CD-ROM)

3. Informal consultation with end users

4. Handouts and supporting documentation for end users

5. Courses and workshops for end users

Although the broadening of the concept of search services in libraries
has many roots, it is clear that one of the major factors behind this trend
is increasing importance of the electronic medium as an information source.
Not that books are in danger of disappearing; but, for certain types of information, particularly in science, technology and business, where there is
a need for rapid dissemination and effective access to new knowledge, the
demand for information in electronic format is growing.

The increasing importance of database searching in libraries is illustrated
by comparing the original *Canadian Standards for Hospital Libraries* published in 1975 with the recent *Standards for Canadian Health Care Facility*

Libraries: Qualitative and Quantitative Guidelines for Assessment, 1989. In the 1975 version, only books, journals and non-print materials accompanied by adequate bibliographic and indexing tools were mentioned as a basis for the provision of reference service (Canadian Standards for Hospital Libraries 1975, 1272). In the 1989 standards, both online search services and support for end users of databases are listed as services that shall be provided, either within the health-care facility or through external sources (p. 15). The standards also contain QA audit quidelines for the function of information retrieval that focus on the provision of MEDLINE searches (p. 39).

A survey conducted in 1985 found that 63% (n=197) of the members of the Canadian Health Libraries Association/Association des bibliothèques de la santé du Canada (CHLA/ABSC) worked in libraries that provided direct access to database searching, and another 33% (n=99) accepted search requests from their users and had the searches run elsewhere (Marshall and Fitzgerald, 1986, 185). A 1989 follow-up survey (Marshall and Park, forthcoming) found that the proportion of librarians providing direct access had increased to 74% (n=221) with an additional 22% (n=66) who had their searches run elsewhere. The percentage of CHLA/ABSC members who provided a variety of services to end users also increased substantially between 1985 and 1989 as shown below:

1. the level of information consultation with end users increased from 45% to 59%

2. handouts or other printed guides for end users increased from 24% to 32%

3. end user training courses increased from 9% to 26%;

4. access to an end user terminal for online access increased from 8% to 13%;

5. provision of CD-ROMdatabases increased from 0% to 20%.

These trends suggest that librarians need to be flexible in their definition of electronic information services and be prepared to change as new user demands and new technologies emerge. Some of the options available to librarians today in selecting database search services include: different kinds of databases (e.g., bibliographic, full-text and numeric); different access routes (e.g., online, CD-ROM and local OPAC); and different kinds of access software (e.g., command language, menus and various types of front ends).

Database searching and reference service

When reviewing approaches to QA in database searching, it is useful to remember that search services are generally considered to be part of reference service. At least some data about searching activities can be gathered in the context of evaluating reference service. The following examples of reference evaluations will be useful to librarians who are interested in the broader issue of reference service evaluation. They also serve as background to the next section of the chapter which deals specifically with the evaluation of database searching.

Shedlock (1988, 49–50) points out the difficulties of defining "quality" in service professions such as librarianship that operate on the basis of personal ideals of professionalism. When it comes to determining quality, librarians tend to rely on the old adage, "I know it when I see it", but measuring this type of quality objectively is another matter. Shedlock states that quality reference service is dependent on three critical elements: the answer, the process and the delivery. The answer must be accurate, the process must be efficient and timely, and the delivery, or style in which the information is communicated to the user, must be positive and service-oriented. Additional useful background on evaluation of reference service is provided by Runyon (1974) who illustrates the library administrator's need for measures of reference and Morgan (1974) who presents the reference librarian's point of view.

There are standards and performance measures for reference service that include basic indicators for the evaluation of database search services or general principles that can be applied to such activities. Schwartz and Eakin's (1986) goal was to establish measurable criteria for the performance evaluation of reference librarians at the University of Michigan. The qualities of librarians that were associated with good reference service were divided into three categories: behavioral characteristics; knowledge; and reference skills. Reference service standards for librarians are provided and indicators, i.e., the behaviours that the librarians should exhibit in order to conform with these standards, are elaborated. Of particular interest to readers of this chapter are the following specific indicators for the evaluation of literature searches:

The librarian is expected to:

    1. advise on the appropriateness of computer searches and alternative databases.

2. provide information on alternative databases.

3. inform new requesters of fee schedules, major research options (time periods, abstracts, online retrieval), and turn-around time.

4. suggest SDI searches. (Schwartz and Eakin, 1986: 6)

Schwartz and Eakin (1986: 8) provide a very useful checklist that includes a variety of reference librarian skills from attitude and demeanor to interviewing, search strategy formulation, knowledge of resources and collections, and knowledge of the particular services and policies of the library.

Judkins et al. (1986) take a somewhat different approach to developing standards for reference services by focussing on the reference product. In their literature review, the authors found that existing standards were primarily quantitative guidelines for different aspects of library services such as collection size and number of personnel. Instead, these members of the Oregon Health Sciences Library Association decided to develop a measure of quality that could be used by librarians in various settings. The reference product was defined as the answer to the reference question, regardless of the format, and six standards that contributed to the quality of the product through the reference process were identified. Although these standards were developed for reference services in general, their applicability to database searching is evident:

1. quality control — the accuracy, completeness, relevance and reliability of the product.

2. appropriateness — determining what is needed and the appropriate amount, level, format and currency.

3. accuracy — ensuring that the information is accurately transcribed, free of typographical errors, collated correctly and copied clearly.

4. documentation — listing sources consulted, search strategy, limitations and identification of all materials given to the user, e. g. full bibliographic citations should appear on all photocopies.

5. timeliness of response — determining when the user needed the materials and evaluating the urgency of the request.

6. accessibility — ensuring the procedures are in place for delivering emergency information.

7. confidentiality — all requests should be treated as confidential, including work forms, log sheets, etc.

8. evaluation — procedures should be set up for ongoing evaluation of reference product by the librarian, peers and users. (Judkins et al., 1986: 38–47)

A review of the QA literature inevitably turns up some useful articles on the complementary topic of performance measurement. This approach takes a systems approach in which a variety of input variables, such as library acquisitions, and output variables, such as the number of books circulated, are used as indicators of the nature, quantity and quality of library activities. McClure and Reifsnyder (1984: 193–94) point out that performance measurement involves establishing library objectives based on user needs, expressing the objectives in quantifiable units and assessing library performance against these objectives. The terminology used in QA is somewhat different. QA directors talk about establishing quality standards, initiating procedures to ensure that the standards are achieved, and, if necessary, taking remedial action. Both approaches, however, have similar goals of monitoring and improving service delivery.

Librarians who are interested in exploring the cost/benefit analyses included in the performance measurment approach will find McClure's article on assessing the quality of reference service through unobtrusive testing useful (1984). McClure suggests four output measures to use as a starting point for assessing the quality of references services:

1. correct answer fill rate;

2. correct answers per reference staff hour;

3. reference services delivery rate; and

4. cost per correct reference answer.

In this section of the chapter, several different approaches to the evaluation of reference services have been reviewed. Each of these approaches can include a component for database search services. A librarian's choice of evaluation method will depend on the resources available for the evaluation and the organizational environment. In organizations where performance measurement of staff is a priority, Schwartz and Eakin's approach would be a good choice. In organizations that are more outcome oriented, the methods of Judkins et al. (1986) and McClure (1984) may be preferrable. The next section of the chapter will discuss evaluation approaches that have focused specifically on database search services.

Evaluation of database search services

Librarians continue to be concerned about the quality of databases and search services. This concern likely reflects the increasing importance of databases and search services in libraries. But it may also reflect a continuing concern with justifying the cost of database searches; a cost which is frequently passed on to the requester. When authors discuss the quality of database search services, the topics covered can be quite varied. A review of the "document record transfer system" developed for the evaluation of online bibliographic systems prepared for the US National Science Foundation suggests why this is the case (Roderer et al. 1981, 3–4). The authors illustrate that for a document to be retrieved online, the following components must exist.

1. document record - a surrogate record that identifies the original document, e.g., a bibliographic citation.

2. document record transfer system - the entire system within which the document records are generated, recorded, transmitted, preserved and used.

3. document record producer - the participant in the transfer system responsible for initially generating and recording document records, e.g., indexing and abstracting services.

4. document record supplier - the participant in the transfer system concerned with recording and transmitting the computer form of the document record, e.g., database vendors such as Dialog and Maxwell Online.

5. document record access point - the participant in the transfer system concerned with retrieving document records, e.g., librarians and other information intermediaries.

6. document record user - the ultimate user of the document record.

Although this model does not fully reflect the current increase in end-user searching and full-text databases, the original model still illustrates the many points at which the databases themselves and the search process can be evaluated. This complexity is also illustrated in Harter's (1986: 107–108) list of 13 main classes of evaluation criteria:

- Coverage
- Size and growth
- Local availability of primary sources
- Currency
- Indexing and cataloguing practices
- Error rates
- Treatment of research
- Record and file structure
- Printing and sorting capabilities
- Cost
- Database aids
- Differences between print and online version
- Review literature

Most of Harter's criteria deal with evaluation of databases at the levels of the producer and supplier. While the features offered by these participants in the document record transfer system are not directly under the control of database users, the review literature that Harter includes among his criteria can influence priorities of producers and suppliers. For instance, Pemberton (1983) calls for some "product recalls" of databases that have quality control problems such as missing words and incorrect spellings. A thorough treatment of this subject by O'Neill and Vizine-Goetz (1988) suggests that error detection and correction methodologies are highly advanced and could be put into place by producers to ensure database quality.

There is also evidence that librarians are going beyond the limits of publicly-accessible databases to improve the quality of access to information within their own institutions through quality filtering. Moore (1989) describes a database of critically-appraised research literature at Texas Tech School of Medicine that resulted from an elective course for medical students. Another paper by Pugh and Moore's (1988) describes a local database at Johns Hopkins University that was created by the librarian in collaboration with faculty and house staff in the departments of neurology, neurosurgery and psychiatry. The database consists of recommended citations with brief annotations to core materials that supported clinical education. A companion, core-experts database lists the Hopkins specialists who contributed to the database.

Chitty and Gelb's (1987) discussion of quality assurance and online searching focuses primarily on the document supplier level. The Quality Assurance
Group of the New England Online Users Group organized a system for track-
ing sources of online access problems among its members and reporting them
to the appropriate producer, supplier or telecommunications network. The
focus of the trouble report form produced by this group was on problems
such as noisy lines, disconnections and slow reponse times.

The majority of attempts to evaluate database search services have been
at the level of what Roderer et al. (1981) refer to as the document record
access point and the document record user. This emphasis is understandable in that these participants in the record transfer system are able to
benefit from and make changes to their own practices as a result of such
evaluations. Studies of the document record access point include quantitative and qualitative reviews of the search services provided by libraries and,
more specifically, studies of the performance of search intermediaries. As
Auster (1986: 193) points out, because of their nature, online services lend
themselves to quantitative measurement. Libraries can record the number
of searches performed, the databases and services used, costs, search length
and the purpose of the search. Information gathered about users can include
a demographic profile, familiarity with database searching and overall satisfaction. Data on the searcher may include the efficiency of the searcher, the
conduct of the negotiation interview, use of search techniques, and interaction with the system and the user. Auster suggests that the problem with
evaluating database searching is not so much with the availability of data
sources, but rather with knowing what to collect and how to use it.

One attempt to bring some uniformity to the evaluation of online searches
by users is the evaluation form developed by the Machine-Assisted Reference
Services (MARS) Discussion Group of the Reference and Adult Services Division (RASD) of the American Library Association (Blood 1983). The group
used four major dimensions of effectiveness of online searches shown below
which were derived from Lancaster's (1977) earlier work on the measurement and evaluation of library services. The Search Evaluation Questionnaire recommended by the group consists of ten questions related to the four
performance criteria and suggestions are made for modifications for different
types of libraries. Suggestions are also made for the conduct of the survey
in different settings. The four performance criteria are:

- Recall - were the search results adequate for the purpose?

- Precision - were the search results relevant?

- User effort - was the search worth the cost, time and effort?

- Response time - was the search completed in reasonable time?

This section of the chapter has pointed out various stages in the production, distribution and use of databases and reviewed some of the major approaches to evaluation that have been developed by librarians. An evaluation of database search services can focus on one or more of these stages. In the past, librarians have tended to focus on the part of the process over which they have the most control, namely the performance of search intermediaries or input/output measures of library search services. Since all of the stages contribute to the quality of database search service, however, it is important to develop an evaluation programme that will address all stages. The work of the American Librarian Association (Blood, 1983) on a standardized evaluation instrument also points out the benefits of cooperation in the area of evaluation. Another helpful approach is for librarians to share evaluation instruments that they have developed. Such a collection of instruments previously used in health sciences libraries to measure both intermediary and end-user services can be found in *Evaluation instruments for health sciences libraries* (Marshall 1990), published by the Medical Library Association.

A sample QA programme for online services

The previous sections of this chapter reviewed some of the efforts that have been made to evaluate reference and database search services. Studies that attempted to assess quality were emphasized. At the outset of the paper, QA was defined as a particular approach to evaluation involving the establishment of standards, initiating procedures to ensure that the standards were achieved and, if they were not, taking remedial action. While this approach has been applied to general health sciences library management (Eagleton 1988; Self 1980) and used in development of the "Standards for Canadian health facility libraries" (1989), its use for in depth evaluation of specific information services is still uncommon. A pioneering article was recently submitted to the Bulletin of the Medical Library Association entitled, "Developing a quality assurance programme for online services" (Humphries and

Naisawald, forthcoming). This paper will be used as a basis for describing how QA can be applied to the evaluation of online search services.

The authors (Humphries and Naisawald, forthcoming) began by listing the basic steps in the QA cycle:

1. Select the subject for review limiting the focus to specific aspects of service that are crucial to offering quality service.

2. Develop measurable criteria based on achievable goals.

3. Ratify the criteria by ensuring that they are relevant, understandable, measurable and achievable.

4. Evaluate the service using the criteria.

5. Identify problems in performance and their probably causes.

6. Implement solutions to the problems.

7. Reevaluate the services.

The authors noted that developing measurable criteria for quality services turned out to be more challenging and complex than they had expected. They examined several studies from the marketing and customer service literature for general criteria that would be appropriate for database searching. The final list included the quality determinants for online service:

- Reliability/consistency/competence/credibility
- Responsiveness/timeliness
- Access/approachability
- Courtesy/communication/understanding customer needs
- Security
- Physical factors

Specific, measurable standards were identified for each of the areas, e.g., for the responsiveness/timeliness dimension, promised turnaround time, priority for patient care and a daily searching schedule were key indicators. The service problems identified in the responsiveness/timeliness area were that, although an informal policy for turnaround time and priority for patient care requests existed, these policies were not advertised or clearly defined for the staff or for users. The solution to the problems was to implement a standard policy of two working days turnaround time, with same day turnaround for urgent patient care requests. Additional procedures were put into place to handle varying search loads and to monitor searching activities. Problems and solutions in some of the other areas were more involved than for responsiveness/timeliness, but followed the same steps in the QA cycle.

The authors reported that the QA cycle had been quite successful in moving the library's database services towards a more professional and customer-oriented program. Many changes were required after the first evaluation, but subsequent re-evaluations proved to be simpler and less time-consuming. Despite the time and effort required to implement this programme over a two-year period, the authors noted that the process did result in a sense of pride, teamwork, and collegiality among the staff members.

Since this was the only report of a specific application of QA to database searching found in the literature, there is clearly much more to be done in the future if QA principles are to be applied to the broad range of intermediary and end-user services. The approach appears to hold a lot of promise for librarians and information specialists who have a keen interest in developing measurable criteria and who are willing actively to use identified problems as a basis for positive change.

References

Auster, E, ed. (1986) *Managing online reference services.* New York: Neal-Schuman.

Blood, R.W. (1983) Evaluation of online searches. *RQ,* **22**, 266–277.

Canadian standards for hospital libraries. (1975) *Canadian Medical Association Journal,* **112**, 1271–1274.

Chitty, M. and Gelb, L. (1987) Quality assurance and online searching. *Online* (2), 110–112.

Eagleton, K.M. (1988) Quality assurance in Canadian hospital libraries — the challenge of the eighties. *Health Libraries Review* **5**,145–159.

Harter, S.P. (1986) *Online information retrieval: concepts, principles and techniques.* Orlando: Academic Press.

Humphries, A.W. and Naisawald, G. (Forthcoming) Developing a quality assurance program for online services. *Bulletin of the Medical Library Association.*

Judkins, D.Z., Hewison, N.S., MacWilliams, S.E., Olson-Urlie, C.O., and Teich, S.. (1986) Standards for references services in health sciences libraries: the reference product. *Medical Reference Services Quarterly,* **5**, (3) 35–49.

Lancaster, F.W. (1977) *The measurement and evaluation of library services.* Washington, D.C.: Information Resources Press.

Marshall, J.G., compiler. (1990) *Evaluation instruments for health sciences libraries.* Chicago: Medical Library Association.

Marshall, J.G. and Fitzgerald, D. (1986) Health sciences libraries as sources of training and support for online physicians. *Bibliotheca Medica Canadiana,* **5**, 184–187.

Marshall, J.G. and Park, L. (Forthcoming) A follow-up study of end-user services in Canada. *Bibliotheca Medica Canadiana.*

McClure, C.R. (1984) Output measures, unobtrusive testing and assessing the quality of reference service. *Reference Librarian,* **11**, (Fall/Winter), 215–233.

McClure, C.R. and Reifsnyder, B. (1984) Performance measures for corporate information centers. *Special Libraries,* **75**, 193–204.

Moore, M. (1989) Battling the biomedical information explosion: a plan for implementing a quality filtered database. *Medical Reference Services Quarterly,* **8**, (1), 13–19.

Morgan, C. (1974) The reference librarian's need for measures of reference. *RQ,* **14**, 11–13.

O'Neill, E.T. and Vizine-Goetz, D. (1988) Quality control in online databases. *Annual review of Information Sciences and Technology,* **23**, 125–156.

Pemberton, J. (1983) The dark side of information — dirty data. *Database,* **6**, (4), 6–7.

Pugh, W.J. and Moore, G. (1988) Psych/neuro core concept database: a quality-filtered database. *Proceedings of the Ninth Annual Online Meeting, New York.* New York: Learned Information. pp. 333–36.

Roderer, N.K., King, D.W., Wiederkehr, R.R.V., and Zais-Gabbert, H. (1981) *Evaluation of online bibliographic systems.* Rockville, MD: King Research.

Runyon, R.S. (1974) The library administrator's need for measures of reference. *RQ* **14**, 9–11.

Schwartz, D.G. and D. Eakin. (1986) Reference service standards, performance criteria, and evaluation. *Journal of Academic Librarianship,* **12**, 4–8.

Self, P.C. (1980) A quality assurance process in health sciences libraries. *Bulletin of the Medical Library Association,* **68**, 288–292.

Shedlock, J. (1988) Defining the quality of medical reference service. *Medical Reference Services Quarterly,* **7**, (1), 49–53.

Standards for Canadian health care facility libraries: qualitative and quantitative guidelines for assessment. (1989) Toronto: Canadian Health Libraries Association/Association des Bibliothèques de la Santé du Canada.

Quality assurance and collection evaluation

Margaret Haines Taylor
Head of Library and Information Services,
King's Fund Centre, London, England

Introduction

Quality assurance programmes in hospital libraries should review the performance of all aspects of the library service. The previous chapter pointed out that while evaluation of reference services and online activities is not new, the application of QA principles to database search services is a recent development. Similarly, collection evaluation has been a regular activity in libraries for years but its inclusion in a hospital-based quality assurance programme dates only from the 1980s.

Collection development activities are critical to the success of other library services because they give rise to the resources by which other services are provided. Thus, they should be, and usually are, among the first areas of library service to be assessed. Most librarians who are confronted with the prospect of developing a QA programme for the first time are relieved to find that they have already been engaged with audit-type mechanisms for years simply because of their collection evaluation activities.

The QA plan co-ordinates and rationalizes evaluation activities in all areas of the library into a strategic plan which:

- sets priorities within services for evaluation;

- determines the standards by which the collection or other service will be measured, thus determining the method which is most appropriate to the evaluation;

- relates the results to the original goals of the library;

- takes the evaluation one step beyond measuring performance by recommending solutions to the problems demonstrated; and

- sets in process the necessary follow-up evaluation activities to see if improvements have followed the introduction of the solution. (Self and Gebhart, 1985)

The results of the QA programme in the library are also fed into the hospital-wide QA activities so that improvements or problems in library service delivery can be identified as contributing to the overall success or failure of the hospital in improving services to its patients. The placement of the results of the library QA programme within the overall hospital QA activity is a very important difference between most library evaluation and that which forms part of QA. It usually means that results of QA evaluation exercises are taken more seriously by hospital management than if they are shown as a separate library evaluation exercise.

In this chapter, my experiences with QA and collection evaluation at the Children's Hospital of Eastern Ontario in Ottawa, Canada, and more recently in the King's Fund Centre in London, England are reviewed. These two very different situations have taught me valuable lessons: that using a quality assurance approach with collection evaluation can maintain quality of services in a period of retrenchment in the first case and that collection evaluation can be used to set the baseline for quality assurance activities in the latter case. Before I elaborate, however, I shall briefly review the collection valuation methods commonly used in hospital libraries and, in particular, in QA programmes so that I can make reference to these methods later.

Collection Evaluation in Hospital Libraries

Writers on collection development agree that the key stages are: policy development; selection and acquisition of materials; evaluation of the collection; and, sometimes, deselection. Collection evaluation is only one stage in this process but it is critical to the success of the others. It can determine whether the selection and acquisition practices accord with the library's mission. It can also determine whether the policy actually meets user needs. It can demonstrate how well the library is doing in comparison to other libraries. It can give a more accurate picture of the scope and depth of a collection and can identify strengths and weaknesses. Collection evaluation is thus an essential management process which helps one to assess and improve the quality of a library collection.

One of the ways collection evaluation methods are categorized is client-centred vs collection-centred (Bonn, 1974) Collection-centred methods focus on the size, depth, scope and significance of a collection usually in relation to standards developed by a professional body or to a standard bibliography written for a certain type of library. The assumption is that there is a direct relationship between the collection that scores well on these methods and user satisfaction (Faigel, 1985). Methods include compiling statistics, checking core lists, and direct evaluation by experts.

There have been many references in the literature to the collection-centred approach in health libraries (for example, Kronick and Bowden, 1978; Day et al, 1979; Gallagher, 1981). Core-list checking is a favoured method, arising from the popularity of the Brandon list (Brandon, 1987), the Checklist for Nursing Libraries (South West Thames Regional Library Service, 1985), etc. This method has often been used in quality assurance plans to introduce measurable criteria into assessing a collection against an otherwise vague standard of collection quality. For example, a standard may state that a library must have an "adequate" collection for the staff in a hospital of a certain size and the library staff may decide that this standard is met if the library has a certain percentage of titles that are on a professionally accepted core list of titles.

Client-centred methods try to reduce the subjective judgments on collection adequacy by measuring the interaction between users, the collection, and the systems the library has designed to facilitate use of the collection, i.e., the utility of the resource (Hall, 1984). Common client-centred methods include circulation and journal use studies, accessibility and availability studies, interlibrary loan analyses, and user surveys.

Favoured client-centred methodologies used in health libraries include journal evaluation studies (Bastille et al, 1980; Byrd et al, 1978) especially those which also survey users about the collection (Ash, 1977; Bess, 1978; Trainor, 1986). The problem in using these methods in quality assurance programmes is in deciding what constitutes an accepted standard of use for a journal title. There are good examples of standards for health libraries which include suggestions on the number of journal titles for a given size of library, but how to relate this type of standard to use statistics for any particular library is less obvious. Generally, a librarian must develop her own criteria of what constitutes adequate use of a journal by the library's clientele.

Other collection evaluation methods such as citation analyses, interlibrary loan studies and cost-effectiveness studies have also been reported in the literature (Hafner, 1976; Byrd et al, 1982; Kraft et al, 1976). The use of a cost-effectiveness methodology in a QA programme is described below.

Collection Evaluation At CHEO

The Children's Hospital of Eastern Ontario is a tertiary care pediatric hospital serving a population of about 500,000 in Eastern Ontario and Western Quebec. The CHEO Library has been in operation since 1974 and serves the needs of all hospital staff: medical, nursing, allied health, ancillary and administrative staff. The Library has always been active in evaluating its services, particularly use of its collection and user satisfaction with interlibrary loan and online searching services. However, the evaluations conducted in the early years of the CHEO Library were not related to other hospital evaluation activities until the advent of the quality assurance programme in the early 1980s.

In 1981, the Quality Assurance Committee of the Board of Trustees of CHEO was established with the mandate to "receive and discuss all matters related to quality of care and ensure that mechanisms are in place to monitor and assess the quality of that care". The QA Committee's attention was primarily on clinical care departments and on issues such as medical ethics and confidentiality of medical records. The Library's involvement with this Committee was minimal until 1983 when the Canadian Council for Hospital Accreditation required all departments in Canadian hospitals to formally and officially establish procedures to evaluate the quality of their services and performance of their personnel: in other words, to have a QA plan in each department. This is when my experience with QA began.

I followed the procedures outlined above in my introduction: I developed standards for each of the objectives I had previously set for the Library in line with the Library's mission statement. I then developed measurable criteria for these standards and performed regular audits of our services to see how we were performing against these standards.

The first QA audit in the Library centred around the book stock because book buying had been declining in recent years. The core-list checking approach was adopted, but as no core-lists existed for pediatric libraries at the time, the Brandon List was used, as it was a well-known and professionally accepted core list for a small medical library. The criterion chosen to demonstrate our performance in meeting the standard of providing an adequate book collection was the number of titles on the Brandon list and the percentage compliance chosen for this criterion was 80%. In fact, after checking the collection against the list, the library was found to have only 19%.

The reason suggested for this low compliance was an inadequate resources budget which had been eaten up by increased journal costs. The solution proposed was a $10,000 grant to augment the book stock. This proposal was supported by a graphing approach to collection analysis which had been suggested in the literature (Pedersen, 1986). A bar diagram was produced which showed the collection strengths in number of volumes for each major Library of Congress classification group, e.g., RJ, RK, etc., and within each bar, the percentage of titles over five years old. As most bars showed very small percentages for new titles, it supported the core list checking audit. This QA audit proved successful in demonstrating the need for additional funding for book resources and the grant was approved. I had never before been able to have my requests for increased book funds taken seriously by administration and I was impressed that this time, having the "negative" outcome presented to the QA Committee and ultimately to the Board of Trustees meant that something was done!

This audit, as with most of those done in the CHEO Library, was chosen because a particular goal was identified as a priority for assessment. However, audits were also done when "critical incidents" or problems arose. For example, not long after the book collection audit, the hospital announced major budget cuts and I was asked to make substantial savings in staff and collection resources: from 6% initially to 20%. I concentrated on the journal collection, as the book budget was still a very small percentage of the total resources budget. As the issue was cost savings, an audit focusing on cost-effectiveness of the collection was carried out. Using the QA approach, the journal collection still had to meet professional (Canadian Standards for Hospital Libraries, 1975) and also our own standard which stated that the collection must represent current interests of the hospital staff. I also added into the equation that these titles must be provided in the most cost-effective way, i.e., the **cost per use** of a given journal could not be higher than the **cost to borrow** an article from that journal on interlibrary loan. Thus, the real cost of interlibrary loans including staff costs had to be established and each journal had to have a cost per interlibrary loan and a cost per use developed. The interlibrary loan cost had to be calculated in relation to each library that lent materials to CHEO.

The cost of getting an article on interlibrary loan from a particular library was based on the cost of borrowing an average length article (nine pages) and the average amount of time a staff member spent on interlibrary loan activity (e.g., locating items and photocopying). For each of the 400 journals in the collection, the least expensive interlibrary loan location was identified and the ILL cost for each title established. The use for each journal (based on photocopying, in-library use, routing and circulation statistics) was averaged over its lifetime at CHEO and the current subscription cost was used to produce a cost-per-use figure.

Over 100 journal titles were identified as possibly not cost-effective to purchase. I informed Administration of these findings and of the potential savings that would result from cancellation of these titles, but I pointed out the negative consequences of this action. Not having these journals in the library would reduce the likelihood that health professional staff would be aware of their contents and, thus, they would be able to request articles on interlibrary loan. This would potentially limit their professional knowledge. Also Library staff would be spending far more time on clerical work than on direct reference service to users. Furthermore, some libraries would be annoyed by the increased interlibrary loan demands from CHEO and might raise their ILL charges, etc. Unfortunately, the journal cancellation project continued.

To help in the cancellation process, we surveyed all departments with the list of library journal holdings, and the list of cancellations, asking for comments on the impact of cancellations on the work of the staff and asking for rankings of preferred journals. This resulted in a revised cancellation list which did not include any core medical titles (i.e., Lancet, JAMA, BMJ, etc), pediatric titles, or any titles which the departments rated as a priority. The savings from the cancelling amounted to $13,000 which, together with some savings in temporary staffing, achieved a total library budget cut of about 20%.

A follow-up evaluation to determine the impact of the cancellations on the collection goals and on other library goals would have been the next step in the QA cycle but I could not undertake this as I left CHEO in 1988. However, the QA process:

- had demonstrated that I had worked through this problem in a very systematic and thorough manner using accepted methodology and standards;

- had helped me involve other staff in the hospital in the process and thus showed them that their opinions were vital in this process;

- had indeed delivered considerable savings to the Administration;

- yet had placed the onus for the potential negative outcome of the Library's budget cuts with the QA Committee and the Board.

I doubt that we would have fared so well, given the severe financial crisis the hospital was in, if we had not had the "protection" of the QA plan.

To summarize the experience with QA in the CHEO Library overall, it was hard work, frustrating, challenging, edifying and satisfying. It was also the first time that library evaluation activities had received so much attention from Senior Administration and the Board. As an American colleague has written; the QA process is a useful public relations tool and a way to educate management about the service priorities in libraries (Fredenberg, 1984).

Collection Evaluation at the King's Fund Centre

The King Edward's Hospital Fund for London is a leading independent charity involved in improving health care by assisting hospitals and other agencies. One of the operating arms of the Fund is the Centre for Health Services Development which includes a library offering a comprehensive information service on health care policy, planning and management. The users of the library include a wide range of people working in the health service; students in health administration, nursing, hospital building and design, and public health; journalists and market researchers as well as staff.

Three factors were catalysts for a collection evaluation project in this library. First, the library was experiencing major difficulties because no formal collection policy existed and the practice had been to try to collect everything related to management of health care except clinical materials. As budgets did not allow the acquisition of sufficient non-clinical materials, the library was getting further and further behind in acquiring new material. A new and well publicized collection policy was needed which would take into account the mission of the King's Fund Centre and the availability of other specialist health management collections, thus narrowing the collecting practice of the Centre Library. Moreover, the collection needed to be assessed against this policy to facilitate appropriate weeding.

The second factor leading to collection evaluation was the imminent implementation of an automated library system. All items in the collection had to be bar-coded in preparation for automation and thus it was important to weed from the collection those items which were out of date or irrelevant to avoid unnecessary handling of materials.

A third factor which moved us towards evaluation was the plan to develop a quality assurance programme in the following year. The King's Fund Centre actively promotes quality improvement in health services: I am trying to develop evaluation programmes focussed on improving the quality of services delivered directly to library users at the Centre and indirectly to the NHS through the provision of information to health service managers.

The collection evaluation project had three distinct phases. The first phase was to decide subject coverage and mandate. I had already developed a mission statement, and key objectives as part of a forward plan and one of my key objectives was to rationalize collection development activities. I embarked upon this by consulting all senior managers to determine subject areas important to their teams' work which were not well covered by the Library. The results of this consultation were reviewed at a Library staff retreat at which we decided that the Centre's policy could be modelled on the American Hospital Association Library's collection development policy, which requires for each subject:

- a definition;

- a level of depth of coverage;

- information on the formats, geographic and imprint coverage for this subject; and

- an indication of the relevance to other subjects in the collection (Library of the American Hospital Association, 1983).

The remainder of the retreat was spent in examining our impression of the collection in terms of:

1. subjects in which the library should collect comprehensively and does;

2. subjects in which the library should collect comprehensively but does not;

3. subjects in which the library should not collect comprehensively but does; and

4. subjects in which the library should not collect comprehensively and does not.

As expected, most discussion centred on subjects in groups 2 and 3.

The draft policy devised at the retreat was then used for phase two of the collection evaluation project: a major subject grading exercise using a modified version of the RLG *Conspectus* approach to collection evaluation. *Conspectus* was developed primarily as a tool for analyzing large library collections in an attempt to facilitate resource sharing and co-operative collection activities (Gwinn, 1983). However, it has also been used successfully in smaller libraries (Buckingham, 1987; Stubban, 1988).

All professional librarians were involved in the project and met several times a week for several months. Prior to these sessions, the librarians had examined the collection to determine the existing collection strength and more appropriate collecting intensity for the subjects discussed at the retreat. During these sessions, each classification code was discussed to debate its definition, existing and proposed depth of coverage and relationship to other classification codes. The depth of coverage was based on the levels used in the *Conspectus* tools, i.e., each subject was given a depth level from 0 (not collected) to 3 (a research level collection). We decided to use four levels instead of the normal six because of the unique nature of the collection. A fifth level (level 4) was used for King's Fund publications as we keep everything published by the Fund regardless of the subject.

The subject grading sessions were often frustrating and tiring as the librarians wrestled with inconsistencies in the use of the classification system, difficulties in relating classification codes to broad subject areas defined during the retreat, and differences in collecting strengths for the same subject in various parts of the collection. It took a total of 200 person hours to complete the first round. Problems caused by wrong classification codes have still to be resolved and new codes created, but the basic work has been done and librarians involved in collection development have a clearer idea of what is in the collection, and a policy on the types of subjects they should be selecting and weeding.

The third phase of the collection evaluation exercise actually took more hours than both the first two combined. This was a major inventory, weeding and bar-coding exercise. It took 705 hours of work over seven days by nine library staff and a few volunteers. Unfortunately, this library could not use any form of circulation statistic to assist in weeding as the collection is for reference use only. The new automated circulation system will accept recording of in-library use and thus future weeding exercises will have useful management data to assist in decision-making. But, for the first weeding exercise, the criteria for weeding became date of publication, physical quality of the item, and current collecting intensity code for that subject.

In 1991 a new quality assurance programme will assess whether the collection continues to support the goals set for the library in line with the mission of the Centre. Standards and criteria used in the QA programme will have to be developed from scratch as no standards or core lists currently exist for unique libraries such as the King's Fund Centre Library which is a combination of a special and a public library. The ultimate challenge for the Centre Library is one faced by all health libraries engaged in quality assurance: it is to facilitate improvements in the services of the parent institution through the provision of better library services.

References

Ash, J. and Morgan, J. E. (1977) Journal evaluation study at the University of Connecticut Health Center. *Bulletin of the Medical Library Association*, **65**, 297-299.

Bastille, J. D. and Mankin, C. J. (1980) A simple objective method for determining a dynamic journal collection. *Bulletin of the Medical Library Association*, **68**, 357-366.

Bess, E. D. (1978) Faculty participation in an evaluation review of low-use journals. *Bulletin of the Medical Library Association*, **66**, 461-463.

Bonn, G. S. (1974) Evaluation of the collection. *Library Trends*, **27**, 265-303.

Brandon, A. N. (1987) Selected list of books and journals for the small medical library. *Bulletin of the Medical Library Association*, **75**, 133-165.

Byrd, G.D. and Koenig, M. E. D. (1978) Systematic serials selection analysis in a small academic health sciences library. *Bulletin of the Medical Library Association*, **66**, 397-406.

Byrd, G. D. et al. (1982) Collection development using interlibrary loan borrowing and acquisitions statistics. *Bulletin of the Medical Library Association*, **70**, 1-9.

Buckingham, J. (1987) NCIP, conspectus methodology and Canadian health sciences collections. *Bibliotheca Medica Canadiana*, **8**, 136-139.

Canadian standards for hospital libraries. (1975) *Canadian Medical Association Journal*, **112**, 1271-1274.

Day, R. A. et al (1979) Comparison of holdings of NLM (CATLINE) with those of resource libraries. *Bulletin of the Medical Library Association*, **67**, 25-30.

Eakin, D. (1983) Health science library materials: collection development. In: *Handbook of Medical Library Practice*. 4th ed. edited by Louise Darling. Chicago: MLA.

Faigel, M. (1985) Methods and issues in collection evaluation today. *Library Acquisitions: Practice and Theory*, **9**, 21- 35.

Fredenburg, A. M. (1984) The quality assurance issue: one hospital library's approach. *Bulletin of the Medical Library Association*, **72**, 311-314.

Gallagher, K. E. (1981) The application of selected evaluative measures to the library's monographic ophthalmology collection. *Bulletin of the Medical Library Association*, **69**, 36-39.

Gwinn, N. E. and Mosher, P. H. (1983) Co-ordinating collection development: The RLG Conspectus. *College and Research Libraries*, **44**, 128-140.

Hafner, A. W. (1976) Primary journal selection using citations from an indexing service journal: a method and example from the nursing literature. *Bulletin of the Medical Library Association*, **64**, 392-401.

Hall, B.H. (1984) Writing the collection assessment manual. *Collection Management*, **6**, (3/4), 4.

Kraft, D. H. et al (1976) Journal selection decisions: a biomedical library operations research model. *Bulletin of the Medical Library Association*, **64**, 255-264.

Kronick, D.A. and Bowden, V. M. (1978) Management data for collection analysis and development. *Bulletin of the Medical Library Association*, **66**, 407-413.

Library of the American Hospital Association. (1983) *Collection Development Policy of the Library of the American Hospital Association*. Chicago: AHA.

Pedersen, W. A. (1986) Graphing: a tool for collection collection development. *Bulletin of the Medical Library Association*, **74**, 262-264.

Self, P. C. and Gebhart, K. A. (1980) A quality assurance process in health science libraries. *Bulletin of the Medical Library Association*, **68**, 288-293.

South West Thames Regional Library Service (1985) Checklist for nursing libraries: checklist 5, reference works. *Health Libraries Review*, **2**, 128-132.

Stubban, V. L. (1988) Use of the RLG Conspectus as a tool for analyzing and evaluating agricultural collections. *IAALD Quarterly Bulletin*, **33**, 105-110.

Trainor, M. A. (1986) Journal evaluation. *Bibliotheca Medica Canadiana*, **7**, 208-210.

Setting inter-library loan standards in a nursing library

Lydia Porter
Information Officer, Quality Information Service,
The King's Fund Centre, London, U.K.

Background to Normanby Library

Normanby Library is typical of libraries which serve schools of nursing in Britain today. It is run by one fully qualified, chartered librarian, who has a full-time unqualified library assistant to provide clerical help. When the library was established, it served the information needs of the student nurses, physiotherapists, midwives, and staff members of the school of nursing. However, over the years, more courses and students have been added to the college, all needing library services. Although each new course provided the library with a book budget, little thought was given to extra staffing, with the result that today, Normanby Library serves five schools (Nursing, Midwifery, Physiotherapy, Radiography, and Dental Hygiene and Dental Surgery Assistants) and the District Training Unit. Clearly, the library cannot now cope with the volume of work which these extra users demand. It is not short of funding to buy textbooks and journals (it has approximately 11,000 books and 80 current journals), but it does not have the staff to carry out the procedures to get the books on to the shelves.

At the beginning of 1989, rumours were spreading that Normanby College was likely to be one of the test sites for the new nurse education system "Project 2000". This meant that future student intakes would be attending

113

the college full-time. With the introduction of Project 2000, students will no longer spend most of their time on the wards, but will be based in the classroom for the first 18 months of the course, with some clinical experience during the final 18 months. For Normanby Library, the introduction of this course could prove disastrous, since a possible 80 students would need to use the library at the same time during the first intake, and an extra 80 for every intake during the following 3 years.

With this thought in mind, the librarian decided to carry out a work-study to identify problem areas of library procedures. By keeping a daily diary, both the librarian and the library assistant were able to monitor those library tasks which were or were not being executed efficiently. The results of the study highlighted, amongst other things, that the inter-library loan service, overdue reminders (and as a consequence of this, book reservations) and book processing (including ordering, cataloguing and classifying) were areas in which delays were having an important impact on the library service.

After the work study was completed, the librarian recommended that:

> "Standards should be set for Normanby Library staff, with a view to ensuring a good quality of service.....The Library staff will then monitor their work: if it is not possible to achieve the standards set, a report will be made to the Director of Normanby College, seeking additional staffing." (Clark, 1989)

What standards?

Setting standards is not a paraphrase of quality assurance. The standard setting exercise is a small part of a total quality assurance programme which is still being developed and introduced into the library.

The library assistant was given the task of setting standards for the three areas mentioned above which were proved to be problematic by the work study: (1) the inter-library loans system; (2) the book reservation system; (3) the book processing procedure. However, it quickly became apparent that for one person to attempt to write three standards at once was a mammoth if not impossible task. The book processing standard was postponed, since the librarian did not feel it was as urgent a task as the others, which were more visible to the library users. Because of staff shortages both librarian and assistant felt that there was not enough time to develop it in sufficient detail before the first intake of Project 2000 diploma students began to study at the college. Consequently the development of standards for book processing was postponed until at least one other member of staff became available.

The library assistant wrote draft standards for the book reservation process, but due to difficulties in recording the necessary data, the monitoring of the standard was not executed accurately enough and it was decided to review that particular standard and the problems which it highlighted at a later date. Consequently, the library assistant's efforts were concentrated on the inter-library loans system.

Inter-library loans

When members of the library need a book or journal which is not in stock, they must request it as an inter-library loan. The service is currently provided free of charge to all full members of Normanby Library. The librarian has two choices: (1) to request the item from the British Library Document Supply Centre (BLDSC); or (2) to request the item through the South East Thames Regional Library and Information Service (SETRLIS), a network of health science libraries within the South East Thames Regional Health Authority. This is a free service for participating libraries.

It is important to note that before the standard-setting exercise, no surveys had been undertaken to ascertain what library users thought of the service. The length of time the process took from users making their requests to actually receiving them had never been accurately evaluated either. Members were usually advised that requests would take up to two weeks; however, there appeared to be no justification for choosing such a random time-limit. Consequently, one of the aims of the exercise was to find out whether the period of two weeks was a correct assumption.

Another objective was to provide a definite framework for the procedure so that a written policy regarding inter-library loans could be formulated. The existence of written standards, procedures and policies would also ease the way for any new member of staff to take on the inter-library loan duties without too much difficulty.

The librarian felt that users of the service were not kept adequately informed of problems which may arise with individual requests. Quite often, the British Library is not able to supply items immediately and informs the requesting library of the reason for the delay. In Normanby Library, this type of difficulty would be logged on the relevant request form, but the user would not always be informed. It was hoped that the standards would be able to solve this problem.

After a long and fruitless search, trying to find references to other libraries which had experimented with similar projects, the library assistant despaired at ever being able to write the standards. Although there are a number of papers extolling the virtue of quality assurance (for example, McFarland, 1985; Fredenburg, 1988; Gebhart, 1980; Kirchner, 1985), none of them provided a simple enough beginner's guide to writing standards. Eventually, the nursing literature was reviewed in the hope of applying nursing techniques to library services. An initial attempt was made using Mason's (1984) book on writing standards, but the results were unsuccessful.

After the standards had been put on trial, a copy of Kitson's, *Steps to Setting Achievable Nursing Standards* (Kitson, 1988) was obtained, and used to guide rewriting of the original attempt. Kitson's work is also used by the members of staff of the School of Nursing in setting their standards.

Standards should comprise a level of performance which is agreed by all members of the library staff and should reflect a level of service which is acceptable to both staff and users, which is achievable and which can be regularly monitored. The standards developed at Normanby Library consist of three criteria:

1. structure criteria are the resources necessary to successfully complete the task under review;

2. process criteria are the actions which the library staff take to achieve certain results; and

3. outcome criteria are the desired effects or results of the service which must be measurable.

The first draft of the standard was introduced on February 13th 1990 and was to run initially for a period of one month. All data were then to be collated by the library assistant, and the standard was to be assessed and re-written if necessary. The draft standard, including all its mistakes can be seen in Appendix A.

The major problems encountered in the first attempt, were (1) the inclusion of a user satisfaction survey, (2) the misunderstanding of the process criteria and (3) the attempted measurement of outcomes which could not easily be measured.

User satisfaction survey

The second structure criterion of the original standard, reads:

> "An inter-library loan history form including details of ... the user's satisfaction with item (measured by questionnaire) is available for each transaction".

Much work has been done recently within the Health Service to measure patient satisfaction. This is an integral part of quality assurance, since it provides feedback from the consumer as to what they think of the service they have received. The attempt to integrate a user-satisfaction survey with a standard-setting exercise was rather too ambitious.

A great deal of thought went into the construction of the questionnaire (see Appendix B), with the aim of measuring users' satisfaction with the items which the library service obtained for them. It was assumed that if students referred to articles or books which had been obtained through the inter-library loans service, then the service had been useful. If users repeatedly made requests, then they must be satisfied with the service.

With hindsight, it seems obvious that it is not realistic to expect one person to attempt to develop achievable standards, survey user satisfaction and continue to execute daily tasks essential to the smooth running of a library service, all within the space of a few months. It is still hoped that a more detailed survey of the use of and satisfaction with the inter-library loans service will be undertaken. In fact it is an essential part of assuring the quality of the service, considering that before the current exercise, no users' views had been incorporated into the procedure.

Each person who had requested an inter-library loan during the trial period received a questionnaire when she collected the item from the library. One of the difficulties encountered was in preventing users from receiving more than one questionnaire. Most users request several items at a time and although the survey aimed to assess the extent of satisfaction with each individual item, it was soon discovered that filling in more than one questionnaire would become tedious. Consequently, users would either not give adequate details, or would not complete them at all. If the survey is to be done again it must be to evaluate the service, rather than the items it provides.

Although the survey was inappropriately used, it did highlight some interesting facts. Fifty-one questionnaires were sent out and 38 were returned

(74.5%). Twenty-four (63%) respondents requested the item to use in study, which suggests that the service is well used by students. This assumption is also supported by the fact that 21 (55%) users said they made a reference to the item in an essay. Only 5 (13%) people took the opportunity to make comments about the service, and two of these referred to the length of time it took to obtain items. One user felt that some type of acknowledgement slip for the user to keep would be helpful, one requested that the library stock more key texts, and one suggested that teachers should provide lists of recommended books to the library before the students arrived, to enable the books to be obtained and kept on a short loan.

After discussions with the librarian and members of the standard-setting team in the School of Nursing, a decision was taken to assume that users would be satisfied (for the purposes of the standard) if they actually received the item which they requested, regardless of whether it contained the information they expected, or whether they referred to it in an essay.

Process criteria

One of the major difficulties with writing standards is understanding the jargon. It is essential when writing standards for the first time, to consult someone who has already done it. Normanby Library standards were written with very little consultation and consequently, some of the criteria were inappropriate. In the original draft standard, the process criteria were confused with the procedure carried out by library staff to procure an inter-library loan for a user. The second attempt at writing standards rectified this fault. (Appendix C)

Kitson (1988) describes process criteria as relating to "the actions undertaken by staff in order to achieve certain results". They would include assessment techniques and procedures, intervention patterns, using documentation systems, patient (user) education and evaluation activities amongst others. Gillespie (1985) is less lucid with a definition of the process as "what goes on in the library; the work of technical and public services". In short, the process criteria are those things that must be done to monitor the standard, not that which must be done to carry out a procedure.

Outcomes

The outcomes of the standards must be measurable. In the draft standard, it proved impossible to measure such things as user satisfaction accurately. Retrospectively it seems obvious that the library could not possibly hope to measure the improvement in a student's ability to write essays (see Appendix A, outcome no. 2b). This would mean plotting the student's work from beginning to end of their study, and even then it would be impossible to ascertain that the service provided by the library was part of the process of improvement, if indeed one could effectively prove an improvement in the first place.

Results

One of the most useful procedures which the exercise involved was monitoring the time it took for a request to go through the system. By keeping a history of each request, the library assistant was able to trace dates of request and arrival, as well as monitoring any delays of which the library was notified. The mean number of days from users handing in the request to them being notified by the library that it was available was 22.5. This showed that the two-week rate the library had previously assumed, was at least one week out. Users were consequently told that all inter-library loans would take at least three weeks.

Although this appears to be a drop in the quality of the service, in reality it is not. If users are promised delivery dates which the library does not meet in the majority of cases, most users would be dissatisfied. If, as a consequence of the exercise, all users now expect a longer wait for their requests, the majority of items will be obtained within the time limit, therefore fewer users will be dissatisfied. This is not to say that the library should not try to improve the speed with which inter-library loans are processed, and in fact this is something on which the library can now concentrate.

The majority of requests took six or seven days from leaving the library to being sent back to the library. This means that most requests were kept in the library for up to two weeks, either before they were processed, or after they were supplied. This was totally unacceptable, and the rewritten standards include time limits for dealing with requests. This particular type of outcome is something which each library must deal with as it thinks fit. In the case of Normanby Library, it has been an unwritten policy to send out inter-library loan requests only once a week. This is unfortunate for the user who submits a request on the day after the previous batch has been posted. However, it is reasonable to expect the library staff to notify users as soon as items arrive in the library.

Since a record was now kept in the way of an inter-library loan history form (a list of dates concerning each item written on to the back of the form on which users submitted their requests), it was now possible to monitor problems and delays. The British Library informs libraries by post of any requests which they cannot immediately supply. This information was not routinely passed on from Normanby Library, with the result that users were badly informed about their requests. After the trial period, a multi-purpose letter was devised, which could be sent out to users to inform them of any problems. This system seems to be working well.

An indirect consequence of the standard-setting exercise was that post was opened more rigorously every day in the library. Previously, if the librarian or assistant was busy with enquiries all day, it was left unopened until a convenient time, which could often be the following day. As a result items could be mislaid. Since it was important to monitor the date on which the requested articles arrived in the library, it became necessary to open the post every day. Fewer items are now mislaid, and urgent requests can be dealt with immediately as a result.

Another important aspect which the exercise highlighted was the need to define the library users. Students at the college, members of college staff, all nursing staff employed by Camberwell Health Authority, plus various paramedical staff, are entitled to become members of Normanby Library. However, the library is also available as an information source for medical students and students of the Institute of Psychiatry, amongst others. It has been the policy of the librarian to offer the inter-library loans service only to users who are entitled to full membership. This necessitated the draft standards to be rewritten changing the word "users" to "members" throughout. It is also clear that a full written policy of entitlement to membership must be devised soon, if policies for library procedures are to be effective.

Conclusion

The standard-setting exercise was useful in a number of ways. Primarily, it enabled the library to identify problem areas in the inter-library loan system, such as length of time the requests are kept in the library before users are notified of their arrival. The project also allowed the staff to keep a close check on the progress of all requests which led to the development of a better communication system between staff and users. By identifying the problems, solutions can be designed and written into the revised standards. Obviously, when the revised standards are monitored, new problems may be discovered, and so the improvement process begins again. This idea of constant monitoring and improvement is one of the essential facets of any quality assurance programme, and should result in an improved service to users.

A further advantage which developed through the exercise was a more thoughtful observation of the purpose of the library. In setting standards, the library assistant had to construct phrases carefully in order to explain accurately the aims and objectives of the inter-library loans system. This thought process enables people to view their tasks with more professionalism and to develop policies which will be in line with the overall aims of the organisation. It should also bring about a more "user-centred" service.

With the initial work study and the following standard setting exercise, the profile of the library was raised considerably. An exercise such as this shows the library in a more professional, businesslike light. In the current atmosphere of cost-cutting and service justification, this can only be to librarians' advantage. By using a technique which is recommended by the organisation, the library is also perceived to be more knowledgeable about the issues which affect its users. The exercise allowed an easy access route to maintaining relations with the teachers of the college, since the library assistant had to set up meetings and talk to the tutors in order to tie in the library's standards with those of the school.

In conclusion, the work is far from finished; it has just begun. Now that standards for one procedure are up and running, there are others to be set, particularly in the two areas mentioned at the beginning of this chapter: book reservation and book processing. Once the standards are set, policies for each process need to be written and reviewed regularly, and this is the stage at which Normanby Library stands. Written policies concerning the inter-library loan service must be available for all members of staff to consult, and to show a more professional face to management. Various problems which need to be addressed are: who is entitled to a free inter-library loan service, who should pay, should the number of requests per member be limited, etc?

Standards are an essential part of the quality process, and can be advantageously employed by anyone thinking of introducing quality into a library.

The Normanby Library experience was a rocky and tortuous journey, littered with pitfalls, but will hopefully prove a useful reference point for others considering embarking on a similar project.

References

Clark, K. (1989) *Work study - Normanby College Library.* (Unpublished)

Fredenburg, A.M. (1988) Quality assurance: establishing a program for special libraries. *Special Libraries,* Fall 277–284.

Gebhart, K.A. (1980) A quality assurance process in health sciences libraries. *Bulletin of the Medical Libraries Association,* **68**, 288–292.

Gillespie, S.A., (1985) Do's & dont's: or points to consider when designing a library quality assurance program. *Bibliotheca Medica Canadiana,* **6**, 187–191.

Kirchner, E. (1985) Quality assurance at work: improving library services. *Dimensions,* January, 26–27.

Kitson, A. (1988) *Steps to achievable nursing standards.* London: Royal College of Nursing.

McFarland, L. (1985) QA: a personal perspective. *Bibliotheca Medica Canadiana,* **6**, 182–186.

Mason, E.J. (1984) *How to write meaningful nursing standards.* 2nd ed. New York: Wiley.

Appendix A Normanby Library Standards: March 1990

Standards for the procedure: obtaining inter-library loans for users.

Primary objective: To procure items for the user which are not in Normanby Library stock.

Secondary objectives:
1. To procure items of use to the user.
2. To assist users in their search for information.

Structure

1. The procedure for requesting loans and photocopies from other libraries is known by the staff.

2. An inter-library loan history form is available for each transaction. It includes details of:

   - date item is requested
   - date request is posted
   - date item is received in the library
   - date item is sent to user
   - user's satisfaction with item (measured by questionnaire)

Process

1. Assist the user in choosing material.

2. Ensure the requests are submitted as early as possible.

3. Deal with urgent requests immediately.

4. Deal with all requests within 1 week of submission.

5. Request items by post from other libraries:

   - a. Check availability of item.
   - b. Complete regional/BL request form.

- c. Send regional requests by 2nd class post.
- d. Send BL requests by 1st class post.
- e. Attach user request form to customer copy of BL form.
- f. File user request forms in request box.

6. Note items in statistics book as they arrive.

7. Notify the user of any problems.

8. Send items to user within one day of arrival in Normanby Library.

9. Refile user forms.

10. Check that user has found item useful.

Outcomes

1. A wider source of information is available to the user.

2. The user will make use of the information, for example :

   a. The user carries out her job more efficiently.
   b. The user writes a better piece of work.
   c. The user supplements her knowledge.

3. The user is encouraged to seek more information.

4. The user will return to the library for further information.

Appendix B: User-survey questionnaire

PLEASE HELP NORMANBY LIBRARY TO PROVIDE A BETTER SERVICE TO YOU BY FILLING IN THIS SHORT QUESTIONNAIRE !!!

All information received will be strictly confidential.

ILL/book number ....

1. Why did you request this book/article?

   - essay/project/study/seminar
   - work interest
   - personal interest
   - other (please specify) ....

2. What date did you receive this book/article? ....

3. How much of the book/article was relevant to you?

   none ... up to 25% ... 26%-50% ... 51%-75% ... over 76% ...

4. How much of the book/article did you read?

   none ... up to 25% ... 26%-50% ... 51%-75% ... over 76% ...

5. Please tick the phrase(s) which apply to you (you may tick more than one) :

   I made a reference to this book/article in my essay
   The book/article gave me something to think about
   I would like to find out more on this subject

I will put the ideas of this book/article into practice
The book/article arrived too late to be of use
The book/article did not contain the information I expected
The library staff did not keep me informed about problems
Other (please specify)........

Please add any comments which you feel may improve the inter-library loans/book reservation service of Normanby Library (continue on the other side if necessary).

Thank you for taking the time to complete this questionnaire.

APPENDIX C: Library service: Camberwell Campus
Standards for library staff - May 1990

Topic: User services
Sub-topic: Inter-library loans
Care group: Library members
Locality: Library services, Camberwell Campus

Standard statement:

Library staff will have the opportunity to examine the inter-library loan service through the use of a structural tool.
Evaluation: Every 2 months.

Structure

1. The procedure for requesting inter-library loans and photocopies from other libraries is known by the staff.

2. An inter-library loan history form is available for each transaction.

Process

1. The history forms will be filled in concurrently.

2. The librarian and library staff negotiate meetings at mutually agreeable times to discuss policy and revision.

3. Inter-library loan procedure will be discussed with a view to identify both positive elements and areas of difficulty.

4. Where necessary, strategies for addressing difficulties will be agreed and time arranged for evaluation of outcome.

Outcomes

1. Members receive items as quickly as possible, preferably within 3 weeks of submitting the request.

2. All requests are posted within 1 week of submission.

3. All members are notified of arrival of item within 2 days of arrival in the library.

4. Library staff will be able to identify problem requests and advise members accordingly.

5. The speed with which inter-library loans are obtained can be evaluated.

6. The inter-library loan policy and procedure will be reviewed.

7. Members will have access to material not available in Normanby Library.

Assuring the quality of consumer health information

Robert Gann

Health Information Manager, Wessex Regional Health
Authority, Southampton, U.K.

Introduction

Until recently most measures of performance in health care in the UK have related to quantity, volume and cost of care, rather than quality. Yet the development of the most succesful food and retail chains over the past ten years have been good examples of a preoccupation with quality products and services (Moores, 1986). The experiences of consumers in this commercial environment are beginning to shape their expectations of health care. People's judgements of hospitals increasingly depend not only on the medical and nursing care given but on how long they have waited for an appointment, whether they were treated considerately and courteously, the environment in which the treatment takes place, and the quality of communication and information giving.

Failure on the part of the National Health Service to meet these expectations will inevitably lead to consumer dissatisfaction and, for the more privileged sections of society at least, increasing use of the private sector. The White Paper on the Health Service, *Working for Patients*, seeks to provide a clear focus for improving quality through the separation of purchaser and provider services and the introduction of contracts for care. Health authorities and general practitioners will look increasingly to place contracts with providers who can give assurances on quality of care, not just on costs and volume (Griffiths, 1989, Bowden and Gumpert, 1988).

Health care consumerism

Today we, as consumers, are generally better informed about all aspects of our everyday lives by virtue of education, communications technology, and the work of consumer bodies and pressure groups. Today many traditional institutions, including the medical establishment, are being drawn towards a more open, participative style to maintain their influence. The growing interest in quality in health care is common to most developed countries; what differs is the means by which it is expressed and the mechanism by which it is monitored. Some countries, such as Australia, Canada, and the USA have formal organisations which act as champions of quality, independent of government or health care providers. The British NHS has always been comparatively unregulated whether by statute or by voluntary bodies. Attitudes are now changing, in response to a growth in consumerism in everyday life and as part of a growing consumer led culture in health service management. The question is no longer whether we should make an issue of quality but about who should take the lead in assuring it (Shaw, 1986).

The main statutory mechanism for consumer representation in the NHS is the Community Health Councils (CHCs) which were established in 1974. CHCs have a number of statutory powers and responsibilities. They must be consulted formally on hospital closures or substantial changes in services. They have the authority to obtain information from NHS managers, to visit hospitals, clinics and other NHS premises, and to make recommendations on improvements in services. CHCs operate at District Health Authority level, and have a membership of approximately 20 lay people. CHCs have performed an important function in collecting and publishing information for consumers.

Some of the most useful surveys of consumer expectations and satisfaction have been carried out by CHCs. Many publish guides to local health services; some offer shop-front information centres for the public. Recently the Association of Community Health Councils of England and Wales has published a Patients Bill of Rights (1986). Amongst rights listed are the right to information about treatment and the alternatives, and the right of access to personal medical records. The Patients Bill of Rights has no statutory authority but it serves as a benchmark for the kind of quality care which consumers are coming to expect.

Dissatisfied patients and relatives are increasingly willing to turn to formal complaints procedures and to the Health Service Commissioner ("NHS Ombudsman") who publishes a regular report, detailing complaints. Similarly the annual reports of medical malpractice insurance bodies show that the British public is increasingly prepared to seek redress in the courts (although to nothing like the same extent as in the USA).

Despite the existence of these formal channels for information, monitoring and redress, some of the most effective work in promoting consumer access to good quality health care in the UK has come from consumer organisations and pressure groups. Organizations like MIND:National Association for Mental Health and the National Childbirth Trust have been instrumental in the development of more humane and participative models of care in mental health and maternity services, respectively. Particularly active in the field of quality assurance has been the National Association for the Welfare of Children in Hospital,which has produced a detailed checklist of services and facilities which should be provided in hospital children's units (1989).

Consumer groups have also been active in publishing information for the public about individual health services, with the aim of giving consumers the opportunity of informed choice. The College of Health broke new ground in 1984 with the publication of its *Guide to Hospital Waiting Lists*, now in its fifth edition (College of Health, 1989). The length of waiting lists for surgery is an area of considerable and justifiable public concern (Yates, 1987). There is an awareness that there can be a great variance in the length of lists, even between neighbouring Districts, and opinion polls suggest that a clear majority of patients would be willing to travel to another hospital if it meant receiving treatment more quickly (National Consumer Council, 1989). The information which would allow patients to identify hospitals with comparatively short waiting lists is collected routinely by District Health Authorities and collated centrally by the Department of Health but until the College of Health published its guide there was no way in which consumers could have ready access to this quality related information.

The government is now actively encouraging GPs to "shop around" for treatment and to refer patients to consultants with the shortest waiting lists. If this exercise in consumer choice is to work, GPs and their patients, need access to up-to-date comparative information. The first Regionwide information service on waiting lists was set up in Wessex in 1988. Called Wessex Waiting Line, the service gives GPs, consumer bodies like CHCs, and patients, access to information on the waiting lists of all consultants in the Region via a phone-in service. The database is updated monthly. Similar services have now been established in Northern Region (using a printed bulletin) and East Anglia (bulletins and an online viewdata service). The argument on whether GPs should be able to advertise their own services has gone on for some time. Now they are being encouraged to produce practice brochures to give patients a more informed basis for decision when choosing their GP.

The development of services like Wessex Waiting Line is an indication of the need for quality related information to enable purchasers of services in the reorganised NHS (be they health authorities or GPs with practice budgets) to select health care providers who meet the right standards of care. Contracts with health care providers will have to specify issues of access, cost and quality. The hardest task will be the specification and measurement of indicators of quality which go beyond input (manpower, money, equipment, etc.) and output (discharge rates, clinic attendances, etc.), to include measures of patient satisfaction and improved health status.

Health care purchasers in the USA (insurance companies, health maintenance organizations, Medicare and Medicaid) have considerable experience of regulatory systems, including the development of sophisticated quality assurance programmes. Managers and researchers on a recent King's Fund fact finding visit (Coulter, 1989) were impressed by the system in New York hospitals. Patients are protected by a bill of rights, dealing with the right to treatment without discrimination; to full information including access to medical records; to ask not to be resuscitated; to refuse treatment; to privacy; to considerate and respectful care; and to a written discharge plan. Several hospitals carry out regular consumer satisfaction surveys and most employ patient representatives to deal with complaints and to ensure patient rights are observed.

Consumer health information services

The experience of health maintenance organizations (HMOs), like Kaiser Permanente in California, suggests that the provision of good consumer information is a key factor in attracting clients to a particular provider. Moreover, those organizations which do provide consumer health information services are particularly likely to attract comparatively young, socially advantaged clients who are likely to require less episodes of care and to be low-cost patients. In turn, the existence of consumer health information and health promotion programmes within a particular HMO should also lead to the adoption of healthier lifestyles, and consequently even lower utilization of services and costs to the provider (Kaiser Permanente, 1987). This recognition of the importance of communication as a crucial element in patient satisfaction has led to many US hospitals producing brochures describing services, and some establishing consumer health information centres or libraries (Rees, 1982).

This movement has been slower to develop in the UK. For some years the only well-developed centres were the Health Information Service at the Lister Hospital, Stevenage and the Help for Health Information Service at Southampton General Hospital in the Wessex Region (Gann, 1986). Over the past two or three years there have been a number of new services set up, characterized by a diversity of settings and funding arrangements. These include consumer health information services based in hospitals (the FACTS information service at Frenchay Hospital, Bristol); in public libraries (Healthpoint in Dorset County Libraries, and Contact West Sussex); in the shopping centre (Health Matters in Milton Keynes, and the Sunderland Health Information Centre); and in the self-help-group support centre (the Nottingham Self Help Team). Services of this kind are still a rarity in the UK but as consumers become more demanding and there is more emphasis on a "mixed economy" of health care, the demand for consumer health information services is likely to grow. And just as the provision of information to consumers is an important element of quality service provision, so must information providers seek to assure their own quality of service.

Looking for models

As consumer health information services in the UK have become more fully developed and sophisticated they have sought to measure their effectiveness against standards of service. But in such a newly emerging area of information work there are as yet few models of good practice in everyday service provision, let alone in quality assurance. One model might be the Citizens Advice Bureau service. Citizens Advice Bureaux (CABx) have been providing generalist information services to the public since 1939, through a network of over 800 CABx dealing with over seven million enquiries a year. Although the independence of each bureau is an important element of the service, each CAB is required by the National Association of Citizens Advice Bureaux (NACAB) to comply with four principles:

- integrity - meaning that the service should not be closely identified with any interest group, should offer a confidential service to enquirers, and should be available to all regardless of race, class or creed;

- accessibility - meaning that the service should be free of charge, available for at least ten hours a week, and should offer equal opportunities in paid or voluntary employment to its staff;
- accountability - meaning that there should be a management committee accountable to NACAB, and clients should have access to their case notes and correspondence relating to them;
- effectiveness - meaning that the management committee is responsible for the effective management of financial and staff resources and for standards of advice work within agreed guidelines. (Citron, 1989)

These are good standards but there is less evidence of work being done on the measurement of whether the standards are achieved. NACAB requires each bureau to make monthly statistical returns through its area offices. These record the topic of enquiry but there are no national client statistics. Confidentiality precludes recording details of the client and as many clients present with multiple problems the enquiry figures do not even give an accurate reflection of the number of enquirers as opposed to enquiries. Most of the available data on client profiles has come from local CAB surveys, which have given more information on the class, age and racial backgrounds of enquirers but very little on their satisfaction with the quality of service received.

By far the most detailed evaluative work on consumer health information provision in the UK has been carried out by the British Association of Cancer United Patients (BACUP). BACUP was launched in October 1985 as a national information service for patients and relatives, the wider public, and health professionals. Information is provided on a free phone line staffed by nurses trained in oncology. Two tools have been used to evaluate the service. An extremely detailed call record form is used to record information about both the enquirer and the nature of the enquiry. Eighty nine coded choices of subject are available, covering site and nature of the cancer, treatments, prevention, counselling and support services. Demographic details of enquirers are also collected unless the nurse considers that this would be inappropriate.

In the first two years over 30,000 enquiries were received (in 1988 22,000 enquiries were received). 80% came from women; 32% were from cancer patients and 39% were from relatives; users were predominantly middle class, and living in southern England. Nearly a third of enquiries related to breast cancer. The call records provide a detailed quantitative measure of BACUP's enquiries; quality is assured by means of user survey questionnaires. The service is confidential so only those enquirers who ask for information to be sent in the post are sent a questionnaire. Questions cover reasons for contacting the service; how easy it was to talk to and understand the nurse; the effects of contacting the service on the mood of the enquirer; and whether any action resulted from contacting the service. During the first two years 6,015 user survey forms were sent out, and 2,827 returned (a response rate of 47%).

While it is likely that those who were happy with the service would be more likely to return the questionnaire, the results were certainly very positive. For example 71% of telephone enquirers reported feeling "much less" or "a little less worried", and only 3% were more worried. The most common actions were to make an appointment with the doctor or to contact a self help group. Eighty nine per cent of respondents described the service as "useful" or "very useful", and 95% said it was easy to understand the information nurse. (Slevin et al, 1988)

In the absence of models of quality assurance in the UK we have, in Wessex, turned to the American experience, and in particular to the Planetree Health Resource Center and Model Hospital in San Francisco. Planetree was created in 1978 to provide a "high touch" balance to the growth of "high tech" medicine in the USA. According to John Naisbitt (1982), whenever new technology is introduced into society, the human response is to counterbalance it with "high touch" or humane equivalents. So recent advances in health care which have brought us organ transplants and genetic engineering have also resulted in hospice care and the birth centre movement. This push for "high touch" is linked to the new wave of health care consumerism, and to a concern with the overall quality of the caring process. Planetree's first step was to create the Planetree Health Resource Center, a health library and information centre open to the general public. The Resource Center provides access to medical and lay health books, as well as information on community resources, self help groups, complementary therapists etc. A "research by mail service" has also been created to accommodate requests for information from people in other parts of the USA.

In 1985 the Planetree Model Hospital Unit was opened. This is a thirteen bed unit, providing care for a variety of medical and surgical patients. The Model Unit encourages patients to be more involved in their care through a variety of learning opportunities which include access to their own medical records; provision of packages of educational materials on tests, medication and treatment; a self-medication programme; stress reduction using relaxation tapes and music; encouraging relatives to stay overnight and become actively involved in the patient's care; and the creation of a healing environment through the design of the unit and the use of "healing arts" (Jenna, 1986).

Research in the USA (and to a lesser extent in the UK) has shown that providing consumer access to health information can have a significant effect on health outcome. Informed patients show higher levels of compliance with treatment, give clearer medical histories, and are more likely to return for follow up appointments (Green 1976). A significant decrease in post-operative pain and complications has also been demonstrated in those patients given access to information (Hayward, 1975). According to Dr John Benson, President of the American Board of Internal Medicine:

> "the humanistic quality of a physician-patient encounter affects the outcome of the patient's problem. The patient's sense of self esteem, integrity, and self respect are increased. Compliance with the treatment regimen improves. Humanism is clearly a parameter of care with psychological implications, not just a nice thing to have." (Benson, 1986)

The humane approach to health care involves the considerate and courteous treatment of patients, good communication and information giving, and a health promoting environment: in short, quality health care.

If patient satisfaction is not only better for health but may also reduce costs, why aren't all patients getting what they want? One problem is that there are no reliable tools for measuring what patients feel is "quality care", including their satisfaction with information given and the uses to which they put it. Detailed evaluation of the Planetree Model Unit by the University of Washington has gone some way towards rectifying this. Questionnaires have been given to patients on admission, discharge, and at three months and six months after discharge, to assess their satisfaction with the care received (including information provision), their health status and social support. The results of these studies are awaited with keen anticipation but indications are that patients who have been treated at the Planetree Model Unit and have had access to information on their own health and treatment compare favourably with control groups on indicators such as patient satisfaction, length of hospital stay and readmission rates (Orr, 1989).

Assuring quality at Help for Health

Finding meaningful measures

Since Help for Health began in 1979 we have kept records of enquiries. For each enquiry received a record form is completed with details of subject of enquiry, type of user (e.g., health visitor, social worker, citizen's advice bureau, member of the public etc.), geographical base, whether the enquiry was received by telephone, letter or personal visit, and the answer given. These data are collated at the end of each month, and then annually. This annual report is then made available to the Senior Manager responsible for Help for Health at Regional Health Authority level (Public Affairs Manager) and to the District General Managers of the client Districts who contribute to the funding of the service.

These statistics have been an invaluable record of the development of Help for Health as the UK's most heavily used generalist consumer health information service. They show a steep and sustained increase in use of the service, by between 15 and 20% every year, to a level of over 10,000 enquiries a year in 1988/89. They make plain the importance of the health visitor as a key information provider as well as consumer; health visitors have been the leading users of Help for Health amongst professionals since the day the service started. It has also been interesting to observe the increasing predominance of enquiries directly from the public, as publicity has become more extensive and effective, and confidence in the service has increased. The enquiry figures have provided an invaluable information base on which to develop publicity campaigns aimed at particular user groups or District Health Authorities. It has not always been comfortable to acknowledge the lack of equity in service provision which sees the people of Southampton Health Authority making forty times as much use of Help for Health as the people of Swindon (4,000 enquiries compared to 100 in 1988/89). Nor has it been easy to justify this situation to the managers of the respective Health Authorities, but at least we have some indicators of areas where improvement can be made.

While our annual enquiry figures have been an important management tool they only provide part of the picture. They give an indication of the "busyness" of the service and a crude measure of output in terms of the number of enquiries turned over in a given period. But they give no real indication of whether the service is providing value for money or whether our customers are satisfied. In part this is because "an enquiry" is not a quantifiable, measurable unit. One enquiry may be answered satisfactorily in a minute ("What's the address of Arthritis Care?"). Another may take a considerable period of research and interpretation of technical information for a lay readership ("What's the latest on Compound Q for treatment of HIV infection, in a language I can understand?").

This was demonstrated quite clearly by research carried out by Kempson into the services provided by Help for Health and by the Lister Health Information Service (Kempson, 1987). It appeared that Help for Health was dealing with a considerably higher quantity of enquiries with similar inputs of staff and other resources. But a closer examination of enquiry figures from the two services showed that while the average length of time spent on an enquiry by Help for Health was 7 minutes, for the Health Information Service it was 63 minutes. Does that mean that Help for Health was providing a more "efficient" service, or that HIS was paying greater attention to quality? Until we have more research it is difficult to say, but the difference may lie in the different characters of the original services. Help for Health has always acted as a clearing house for self help groups while HIS has operated a more literature-based service. It is interesting to note Kempson's observation that the two services are becoming more similar and that between them they offer the best model for the development of consumer health information services in the UK.

In the absence of more sophisticated measures there is a temptation for managers and funders of information services simply to divide the costs of the service by the number of enquiries, and to use cost per enquiry as a measure of value for money. In the case of Help for Health last year this would produce a figure of £3.50 per enquiry. This sounds quite good value but is meaningless without a better idea of what "an enquiry" actually involves. This is, of course, true of all library and information services and not unique to consumer health information (CHI). What is unusual about CHI is the possibility of a particularly close causal relationship between the provision of information and a change in the circumstances of the enquirer. CHI holds the possibility of quite dramatic improvements in health and social welfare, whether this comes through becoming aware of a source of financial help; a change in diet, exercise or other lifestyle factors; identification of a serious side effect of treatment, or a lessening of stress, depression or isolation through contact with a self help group.

Access to information is the essential first step towards these improvements in health status. To assess the real effectiveness of CHI provision we need to be able to measure not only the output of services (the number of enquiries answered per year), but also the outcome (whether our consumers were satisfied with the service provided and, far more difficult, whether there were any improvements in patients' circumstances as a result of receiving the information). In the words of one doctor speaking about the provision of health education leaflets to elderly people, we need to know which pieces of information change lives and which line the cat's box (Rowe, 1984).

A quality assurance plan for consumer health information.

In 1988 Help for Health, in common with other RHA departments including the Regional Library Service, was asked by the Regional Health Authority to develop a quality assurance plan. The plan should include clear, measurable standards with provision for monitoring their achievement. The following standards were agreed:

- the service will respond to requests for information as a priority over all other areas of work;
- the service will respond to all requests for information within 24 hours;
- the service will treat all enquiries in confidence;
- the service will provide accurate, balanced information and will not attempt medical advice or counselling;
- the service will keep information up to date; and
- information will be verified at least annually, and the service will comply with the good practices of the Data Protection Act.

Help for Health's quality assurance plan pledged that the achievement or otherwise of these standards would be monitored through user surveys. Two surveys were carried out during 1988-89. The first (in November 1988) logged every enquiry received over a sample week to ascertain whether the standard of all enquiries being answered within 24 hours was being met. Measuring the achievement of standards on confidentiality, accuracy and balance proved a lot more difficult. However a second survey (of all enquiries received in one week in February 1989) tested levels of user satisfaction, which it was hoped would include these concepts.

The enquiry turnover survey confirmed the findings of Kempson's comparative study of the Lister HIS and Help for Health (Kempson, 1987). Forty percent of enquiries were answered immediately over the telephone in under five minutes. These were mainly requests for the address and details of self help groups. A further 39% were answered in under 15 minutes. These were enquiries answered satisfactorily by the provision of Help for Health information sheets (these have been prepared for over 60 common enquiries) or literature from other organisations held in stock (a core collection of frequently requested material has been built up, with bulk holdings). Twenty percent of enquiries required more detailed research, literature searching etc. In the survey week only two enquiries out of the 188 received were not cleared within the day, either because of the need for detailed research or because of backlog of work. We readily admitted that turnover may have been fast that week because we were being measured; however the similarity with the Kempson findings suggests a reasonably accurate reflection of our everyday work.

This first survey also provided the opportunity to extract other data from the detailed records of time enquiry received and time completed. Monday was the busiest day of the week, closely followed by Friday (particularly Friday afternoons). This is likely to be because people worry about health problems over the weekend and are not able to contact health or information professionals. Similarly the impending weekend may lead to information seeking on a Friday afternoon. We also wonder whether Monday morning information seeking may be due to health panics induced by Sunday newspapers! There is no doubt that more people contact Help for Health in the mornings (in the survey week 67% of enquiries were received between 9 am and 1 pm, and 31% between 1 pm and 5 pm; only 2% were received outside hours by answerphone). It seems that more expensive telephone calls are not necessarily a disincentive when people really want information. In any case, the majority of telephone calls were from professionals who, presumably, were not paying their own telephone bills.

The second survey involved sending a questionnaire to enquirers contacting the service over a one week period. Ideally all enquirers in the week should have been surveyed, but we felt it was crucial not to breach our standard of confidentality in our attempts to measure our achievement of the standards. Like BACUP we were able to send questionnaires to enquirers who gave their name and address in order that we could send them literature. To the others we explained that we were carrying out a survey that week and asked whether they would mind being sent a survey. It was made clear to every caller that they were quite at liberty to refuse. None did so: however, on five occasions Help for Health staff decided not to suggest the questionnaire because it would be obviously insensitive to a distressed or embarrassed caller. During the survey week 122 people contacted Help for Health; 117 questionnaires were sent out and 81 were completed and returned (a response rate of 69%). The questionnaire consisted of a single sheet with 15 open questions, covering satisfaction with the specific information received and the use to which it was put; and attitudes to Help for Health as a service, including whether the enquirer had used Help for Health before, if they had experienced difficulties contacting us, where they would go if we did not exist, and the best and worse things about the service.

Ninety six per cent of the respondents reported that the information was helpful. Of the remaining 4% one replied "only slightly", two "moderately", and one "no". Seventeen respondents classed the information as "extremely useful" and one wrote "I just couldn't have coped without it". Although the questionnaire produced some valuable anecdotal comments about the actual use to which the information was put, it was not possible to trace outcomes in terms of improved circumstances or health status without further follow up. Because of time and resource constraints, as well as confidentiality, this was not done on this occasion. It was clear that many enquirers passed information on to other people (family, friends, patients, clients etc.). A high proportion of respondents (59%) had contacted Help for Health before. This was an encouraging figure as repeat use should be indicative of a level of satisfaction with previous encounters.

Nine respondents reported difficulty in contacting Help for Health. These all related to delays on the Southampton General Hospital main switchboard. Many respondents said that they would have to approach many disparate and time consuming information sources if Help for Health did not exist. This was a welcome response for a service trying to demonstrate its cost effectiveness. This perception was picked up again in the replies to the question on the best thing about Help for Health. Here there were three recurring areas of user satisfaction: the availability and accessibility of a wide range of information under one roof; the speed of response; and the helpful and knowledgable attitude of the staff. The worst thing about Help for Health was equally instructive. By far the most common negative reaction was "not enough people know about it" and publicity could be improved. Other comments related to problems of telephone access and the need for more material to take away.

The results of the surveys were reported to the Regional Health Authority and to client District Health Authorities. We were also committed to act on the findings, and some changes have now been implemented. In particular publicity has been increased with renewed emphasis on our direct telephone line and a loan system has been introduced for books and videos. Our belief in a very broad-based information service has also been reinforced; in both survey weeks enquiries were received on over 100 individual topics.

Looking ahead

In 1990 Help for Health is to leave the umbrella of the Regional Health Authority and will become an independent charitable trust. This is in line with the policies outlined in Working for Patients, regarding devolution of non-core RHA services to districts or independent agencies. A package of information services will then be available to DHAs and other authorities on a contract basis. As we have seen, those clients will want to be assured of the quality of service for which they are paying and this gives a renewed impetus to the search for quality in CHI services. At one level the contract relationship itself should act as a stimulus to quality: if purchasers of information services do not feel they are receiving a good service they will stop buying it. But purchasers will also wish to see quality assurance measures in place before they take out contracts for services. In addition to Help for Health's quality assurance plan, other quality assurance systems are in place or are being developed.

Individual performance appraisal

Most CHI services are small. Typically there will be a single librarian or information officer, supported by a clerical worker or volunteers. In such a situation the objectives of the individual professional are likely to be very close to those of the service as a whole. Many health authorities have now introduced annual objective setting and performance appraisal by a senior manager. Some have introduced performance related pay, linked to the appraisal process. For example, in Wessex, my own personal objectives have included tasks such as:

- boosting promotion of service with the objective of increasing enquiries by 20% ;
- establishing Regional AIDS resource bank by May 1987;
- marketing Help for Health database with objective of creating agreed proportion of budget from income;

  • developing quality assurance plan for service.

Like quality assurance standards, individual objectives should be clear and measurable. There is a tendency for individual performance appraisal to reward new development work without sufficient recognition always being given to carrying out core tasks to a high standard. But in small organisations in particular, where the work of one individual is central to the achievement of the objectives of the service, performance review can be a spur to quality.

Mission statement

Many organisations have developed mission statements which provide a statement of the guiding principles by which the organisation operates. Consumer health information services should be guided by the mission of their parent organisation (health or local authority, charity etc.). The Wessex Regional Health Authority has a purpose: "to ensure that everyone living in the Region has good access to health services of high quality and that people of the Region will enjoy improved health", pursued through a mission based on:

  • performance - to maximise in quantity and quality the current service within the existing capabilities;
  • development - to improve the capability of the service;
  • services - to provide appropriate common services.

In order to carry out its mission the Authority holds to the values of equity, excellence and example.

Within parent bodies, individual services may develop their own mission statements. A good example is the Mission Statement for Health Education produced by the Kaiser Permanente HMO in the USA (Kaiser Permanente, 1987) : "to improve member health and satisfaction by enabling members to be active partners in managing medical conditions, preventing disease, and promoting health in a cost effective manner". A mission statement for a consumer health information service would do well to include some of these essential concepts:

  • equity of access to the service for all potential users, irrespective of class, age, sex, race, physical or mental ability, or geographical location;

- constant development of services to improve the capabilities of information provision;

- example of excellence, given that there are, as yet, few CHI services in the UK and those that there are serve as models for a developing area of information work;

- the overriding principle of enabling consumers to become informed and active partners in their own health care and promotion.

Health outcomes

In consumer health information services we like to think that the information we provide leads to increased knowledge, which in turn produces changed attitudes, which in turn affects behaviour. Studies have shown that this is not always true (Marshall and Haynes, 1983). Behaviour change can precede knowledge or develop independently of it. Information is only one element in the factors influencing behaviour. More than 250 influences on compliance with treatment have been identified, ranging from the weather to safety lock pill dispensers (Haynes, Taylor and Sackett, 1979). The road from the provision of information to a positive health outcome can be a long and rocky one. Consider the example of an information service giving the address of a self help group to a patient. The address may be out of date. The information may be correct but the patient never uses it. The patient may contact the group and receive an unwelcoming response. The response may be warm but, when the patient attends the group, the meeting is hostile or a shambles. The group may be perfect in itself but cater for the wrong age group and the patient may not fit in. And so on.

In trying to assure the quality of CHI services it can be almost impossible to distinguish the effect on health outcome of information provision from the many other factors. "Information is power" is often quoted, particularly by librarians. It isn't: information is only potential power. The growing information overload of everyday life can actually be counter-productive and lead to inertia, apathy and frustration. Information needs to be communicated effectively and people must have the opportunity and resources to use it in their everyday lives. Perhaps the link between information giving and health outcome is too tenuous to measure in a meaningful way but it is worth pursuing. Information may not automatically lead to health, but without information consumers cannot take the first step.

References

Association of Community Health Councils in England and Wales. (1987) *Patients' charter.* London: ACHCEW.

Benson, J. (1986) *The future of the American hospital.* New York: Grantmakers in Health.

Bowden, D. and Gumpert, R. (1988) Quality versus quantity in medicine. *RSA Journal*, April, 333–346

Citron, J. (1989) *Citizens advice bureaux: for the community, by the community.* London: Pluto Press.

College of Health. (1989) *Guide to hospital waiting lists.* 5th ed. London: College of Health.

Coulter, A. (1989) Buyers and sellers. *Health Service Journal*, 99, 1402–1403.

Gann, R. (1986) *The health information handbook: resources for self care.* Aldershot: Gower.

Green, L. (1976) The potential of health education includes cost effectiveness. *Hospitals*, **50**, 57–61.

Griffiths, P. (1989) Quality held in trust? *Health Service Journal*, 99, 1466–1467.

Haynes, R. B., Taylor, D. W., and Sackett, D. L. (1979) *Compliance in health care.* Baltimore: Johns Hopkins University Press.

Hayward, J. (1976) *Information: a prescription against pain.* London: Royal College of Nursing.

Jenna, J. (1986) Towards the patient driven hospital. *Health Care Forum*, May/June, 9–18.

Kaiser Permanente. (1987) *Partners in health: strategic directions for health education.* Oakland: Kaiser Permanente.

Kempson, E. (1987) *Informing health consumers: a review of consumer health information needs and services.* London: British Library/ College of Health.

Marshall, J. G. and Haynes, R. B. (1983) Patient education and health outcomes. *Bulletin of the Medical Library Association*, 71, 259–262

Moores, B. (1986) *Are they being served? Quality consciousness in service industries.* Deddington: Philip Allan.

Naisbitt, J. (1982) *Megatrends.* New York: Warner.

National Consumer Council. (1989) *Consumers and the health service: MORI survey.* London: NCC.

Nation Association for the Welfare of Children in Hospital. (1989) *Quality review: setting standards for children in health care*. London: NAWWCH.

Orr, R. (1989) Personal communications.

Rees, A. (1982) *Developing consumer health information services*. New York: Bowker.

Rowe, M. (1984) Information for health now, with a happy retirement in view. *Health Libraries Review*, **1**,(1), 11–15.

Shaw, C. D. (1986) *Introducing quality assurance*. London: Kings Fund. (Quality Assurance Programme Project Paper).

Slevin, M et al. (1988) BACUP - the first two years: evaluation of a national cancer information service. *British Medical Journal*, **297**, 669–672.

Yates, J. (1987) *Why are we waiting? An analysis of hospital waiting lists*. Oxford: Oxford University Press.

Objectives, standards and guidelines in the Quality Assurance Information Service

Anne Holdich Stodulski
Information Officer, Quality Assurance Programme,
The King's Fund Centre, London, U.K.

Introduction

Today, issues of quality, such as audit, organisational and clinical standards, consumer feedback and participation, and management for quality, are matters of especial debate in the National Health Service. However, examples of qualitative issues have always been open for debate and action in the NHS as shown by the body of literature addressing quality in health care but predating the current debates.

Most people, whether they are politicians, managers, clinicians, support staff or consumers, agree that health services should offer the highest quality care possible within the constraints of costs, available treatments and their benefits for patients, staffing, quality of life and a wide variety of other resource and technological considerations. Especially, it is no longer possible to divorce the highest standards of care and treatment from what is affordable for national health services. As a result, part of the current dialogue in the UK is associated with how "quality" is interpreted, how this influences service delivery and affects the consumer and his/her health care needs.

The Quality Assurance Information Service (QAIS) was established at the start of this debate. The QAIS forms part of the Quality Assurance Programme at the King's Fund Centre for Health Services Development. For more than four years it has been the role of the QAIS to draw together details of activities and publications on all aspects of qualitative issues in health care into a single collection and to disseminate the information to managers, practitioners and other interested groups. This information forms an integral part of DHSS-DATA [1] - the computerised database of the Department of Health Library. The baseline dissemination tool is *Quality Assurance Abstracts* [2] which is produced in conjunction with the Department of Health. In addition the QAIS offers an enquiry service [3].

QAIS objective setting exercise

The QAIS objective setting exercise sprang from a number of closely linked factors including a long standing policy to provide the highest possible quality services to our users within the resources available, and a period of change within the Programme which would have major implications for the shape of future services. Additionally there was a wider exercise to establish goals for the Programme and the development of a mission statement for the Centre.

These changes signalled a new phase for the QAIS, in that during the first years of the service it had been largely a free service operating within extremely limited staffing and resource constraints. However, our relationship with the Department of Health Library and the sophisticated facilities of DHSS-DATA, coupled with the efficient use of word processing and information handling routines within our own microcomputer-based system, had allowed us to press our limited resources to their limits in offering high quality products and services to our users. The new phase of work meant that we would aim to provide a more focussed service to our primary audience, with more user-friendly and valuable services and products. In some areas of our work this would mean introducing fee-based services to users, in others it would mean working closely with members of the Quality Assurance Programme to increase and improve our holdings in key subject areas.

We decided that the wider objective setting exercises within the Centre, together with the preliminary re-shaping of our services for the 1990s, could and should provide an opportunity to build upon the values we held, but which were largely implicit. As a result we spent three months, actively involving the two information workers and the Programme Director, in developing a series of statements that encapsulated not only the current "how, what and why" of the QAIS, but which also took into account the new values and services we wished to offer to external and internal users. This proved to be a relatively painless and short undertaking: our timetable allowed us to devote only one two-hour period a week to developing objectives. The work could have been done much more intensively, but by focussing on one aspect of our work at a time it allowed us to see more clearly how the different elements of the service meshed together.

Like most library and information services, we had some baseline performance and monitoring measures in place. In addition, regular work analysis studies gave an indication of the pattern of work in the QAIS. As many routine elements of the service relied on computer-based processing, some aspects of the work could be relatively easily quantified. Previously our objectives and underlying values were largely implicit. Our immediate purpose in this first examination of our objectives was to make *explicit* statements about our aims and values, and as far as possible, marry them to explicit performance standards and guidelines. Initially the performance guidelines and standards would draw upon upgraded and existing performance and monitoring measures. We recognised quite early on that the standards and performance measures we might use could only be as good as those elements of personal and unit performance that can be measured, and that sophisticated standards can only be built from good basic foundations. We decided, therefore, that our approach to performance measures would be an incremental one, but that all measures must be explicit. Also, all staff of the QAIS should participate in their development because ownership of both personal and unit performance measures would be an important element in their success.

The objectives

As already mentioned, the establishment of objectives for the QAIS took place within a wider context; the development of a mission statement for the Centre and annual objectives for the Quality Assurance Programme. The Centre mission statement (a disliked term for which no alternative could be found) aims to state as briefly as possible the function of the Centre.

Mission statements are highly general statements of purpose whose function is to act as a kind of rallying slogan. The final statement was arrived at by a "top down with consultation" process with all staff of the Centre having an opportunity to contribute to the debate. Programme objectives were easier to develop as each programme has a clearly defined area of interest with several key issues currently being explored. In addition, these could be wordier than the mission statement as they set out the key long-term objectives for the Programme and the specific activities projected for the next 12 months. The QAIS objectives have been produced through a "bottom up" approach with the practitioners setting their own standards, although the input of the Programme Director was seen as crucial to the exercise.

The QAIS objectives follow a pyramidal, three level structure. The apex, or first level, offers a single general statement about the overall objective. The intermediate level contains statements relating to each of the seven main areas that comprise the work and internal and external customer services of the QAIS. The statements at the lowest or most detailed level deal with the processes required for each of the main areas of work as well as performance guidelines and where possible standards of performance that relate to the way the work should be approached or carried out.

We developed this three-tier approach because it allowed us to accommodate objectives dealing with structure, process and outcome. It also enabled us to deal with performance measures and standards in a flexible manner. We envisage that the majority of the seven major objectives will remain fairly stable, and that others may be added from time to time as the needs of internal and external customers change and the subject area itself develops. However, the standards and guidelines are likely to be fairly dynamic, as more sophisticated measures of user feedback, and individual and unit performance are developed.

Standards or guidelines?

The services and work of the QAIS are at different stages of development: for example, *Quality Assurance Abstracts*, our basic dissemination tool, is the most firmly established element of the service and, for a variety of reasons, is likely to undergo little change in the forseeable future; whereas the enquiry service is about to be tightened up and targeted more closely as a fee-based service. We also have two new products: a series of literature reviews and topical highly selected and organised reading lists about to go into production. At this time our challenge was not so much in setting the objectives, but in deciding what kinds of performance measures could be applied to monitoring these elements of the overall service.

LEVEL 1: the following is the primary objective for the service:

> To identify; collect; maintain and disseminate soft and published information about quality improvement in health care, with particular emphasis on information relating to the UK.

LEVEL 2: the following is one of seven statements of objective for the main service elements, four of these relate to outward looking or external user objectives and three are inward looking towards support of internal staff and our own performance as a unit. The objective chosen here is one of the four outward-looking ones:

> The objective of the QAIS enquiry service is to provide individualised responses to requests for information, and to develop the service to become more "user friendly" and "user valuable".

LEVEL 3: the statements at this level have a two-fold purpose. First they focus on the processes and values necessary to provide the seven service elements outlined at level 2, then they state the performance standards and guidelines that will be used to monitor performance. The following examples relate to the enquiry service:

> **Specific objective** - A proper log of enquiries should be maintained that can track enquiries during the process of responding; will facilitate analysis of enquiries and which can be used to identify past users for user feedback.

> **Performance guideline** - An evaluation process should be incorporated into the service that seeks feedback from ALL users not more than three months after their enquiry was completed.

Figure 1:
Examples of the three levels of objective statements

Initially, the debate as to whether to call one's measures "standards" or "guidelines" appears to be merely an issue of semantics. However, it became clear to us that there were very real differences, and that these differences were likely to apply in some degree to any library or information service looking at the services it offers. Once an objective has been identified, performance measures are needed to assess whether individual or unit performance meets that objective. It seemed to us, therefore, that the crucial issue in determining the name of the measure was the extent to which performance could be quantified. If performance could be measured (and it can be for some aspects of service) then we felt that a "standard" could be developed for the service or activity. However, it may not be immediately possible to determine a measure of performance because the activity, product or service is not fully developed, or because the measure relates to the basic values of the service. In such cases we felt that the measure should be called a "guideline". It would thus make explicit a particular approach or value that should be adhered to.

In our objectives we have both standards and guidelines. Standards, as we have said, refer to the more quantifiable aspects of the work: for example, we specify what error levels are acceptable within *Quality Assurance Abstracts*, or how speedily an enquiry should be answered. We have also tried to determine what is practical or possible in achieving the standard. This distinction has been made to emphasise the difference between levels of performance that are practicable: for example, it becomes counter-productive to use limited resources to eliminate every error from a document like *Quality Assurance Abstracts* which follows a regular publication schedule. We believe there is a level beyond which error detection becomes impractical. In addition, financial and resource constraints can often necessitate meeting some standards at a less than ideal level. However, one has to recognise these limitations while striving for the highest standard or level of excellence possible in the circumstances. Indeed it may be worthwhile noting this in the standard in some way.

At present most standards are applied to services aimed at the external customer, whereas our internal customer objectives tend to feature guidelines. This is in recognition of the role we are developing in supporting a rapidly expanding internal customer group. These guidelines express the values we wish to apply to these services and they will change as users identify and develop their information needs. Where standards had been established, for example in relation to quality control, it became apparent, as we refined our new performance measures, that we were actually performing better than we thought, so we immediately made the standard more stringent. In other words, we viewed the situation not as an invitation to perform at a lower level than it was possible to achieve, but as an opportunity to improve performance. On a simple level, standards allow us to compete with ourselves and we hope they will provide guidance on performance for future workers to match or better.

Qualitative or quantitative measures?

It was not difficult to decide that the performance measures aimed for would be qualitative. However, these can be expensive, time consuming and technically difficult to implement, especially for a comparatively new service. Thus, it quickly became obvious that initially most of our measures would be quantitative, largely because this was the kind of information our existing indicators were based upon. Most of our quantitative measures focus on aspects of structure or process, whereas the kind of qualitative indicators we wished to implement would be concerned with outcome and would be based on user feedback. Standards stating that all staff should undertake a period of work analysis to identify daily work patterns, or that enquiries should ideally be dealt with within seven working days are examples of quantitative standards. Other, qualitiative guidelines can be seen in the objectives for our enquiry service: for example, we state that an evaluation process should be incorporated into the service and that all users should be provided with an opportunity to offer feedback within a specific period from their enquiry. As most of our users make their initial contact by telephone, it is particularly important that we should obtain feedback from users. Information workers are accustomed to telephone work but rarely have formal training in interpreting enquirers' needs. Therefore, we set out some detailed supplementary guidance on "how we would wish it done", giving hints and tips on how to get the maximum information from an enquirer without making it seem like an interrogation.

It is our aim to develop a battery of measures for each aspect of the work to provide both quantitative and qualitative information. This will enable us reliably to estimate the cost of sevices, to us and to our users; to look at unit and individual staff members' performance; and to know how our users value the services we offer, how we meet their needs, and how we might develop the service.

Minimal or optimal indicators?

There has always been a debate as to whether standards or indicators of performance should be minimal or optimal/ideal, and both have their place. In practice, many national or broadly applied standards and indicators are based on minimum requirements whilst bottom up or locally developed standards aim for optimal or the best possible performance within local financial and resource constraints.

Our approach in this exercise was pragmatic: in some cases we expressed the minimum level of performance, in others the ideal, and in a number of cases a range of acceptable performance. In future developments of these objectives it is likely that more standards will specify a range of performance. This approach not only recognises variations in individual performance on different tasks, but should also provide a useful tool for reviewing the standard. Where unit performance is consistently superior to the standard, consideration can be given to whether it should be more stringent, and in the case of individuals who also perform better than the standard it may be possible to apply the lessons that the person has learned more generally.

These objectives do not incorporate sanctions for bad performance, but we do make use of target setting and appraisal which should allow worker and manager to examine and adjust performance in a confidential setting. Also, every effort has been made to word the statements in a way that links unit and individual performance because an important part of the exercise was to highlight how closely the two interact and how good or bad performance on the part of the individual can affect unit performance and the performance of co-workers. This last is especially important in a multidisciplinary team like the Quality Assurance Programme.

Examine all or bits of the service?

This was an easy question because, being a small unit dealing in a specialised subject with a fairly well defined primary audience, the areas we work in fell fairly easily into seven broad categories. We had advantages in that we had looked in some depth at bits of the service and the processes they involved and patterns of work before we started. In addition we also had some pre-existing, largely quantitative measures which we could develop. Other measures, like the *Quality Assurance Abstracts* quality control standards and guidelines, had to be developed from scratch. In other libraries and information services it may not be practical or possible to take the "all out" route. Some activities do lend themselves to a modular approach and it may prove best to identify an overall objective for the service plus the main subsidiary objectives together with a timetable of action. We chose to take the "all out" route because it allowed the various modules to be built in a cohesive fashion that will interact and function together as a total system when complete.

What kinds of measures?

As yet, our performance measures are fairly limited and some have been mentioned above. Our ultimate aim, however, is to develop a complete battery of fully operational measures. In addition we have tried to choose measures which minimise the effort of data capture, or where the information needed is a by-product of the administration of a service. For example, the enquiry service administrative database can generate information on:

- the time taken to answer enquiries;

- predicted and real income from the service;

- details of sales of other information products; and

- the amount and kind of work done for enquiries.

It provides regular updates for the team on income and subjects requested and will shortly be used to facilitate user feedback mechanisms. Our quality control measures, unlike those for the enquiry service, are not an administrative by-product but are collected independently of the work of editing and producing the bulletin and are currently being drawn together into a more cohesive whole. The next area we will be seeking to improve will be information about costing of services and cost recovery. This will prove much more of a challenge as so much of what we decide to do will have to take account of the Centre Information Strategy currently under development.

Benefits and disadvantages

When we had set our objectives and identified our performance standards and guidelines we felt that the exercise had had massive benefits and few disadvantages. However, we recognised that we had an advantageous start in that we already had a fairly strong philosophy of service and a value base. Also, we started with an open and analytical approach to our work and, most valuable of all, we all felt motivated to carry through the exercise. This may not always be the case, particularly in larger units where the professional culture and values are less clearly defined and where it may be difficult to involve all the staff in the exercise. In these cases, if the senior information professional does not feel able to act as facilitator, it may be necessary to bring in outside help: for example, a quality assurance professional or a quality circle facilitator. There is also a definite time cost in the initial stages with which some units might not be able to cope. Whilst we were prepared to find the time to undertake an extensive review of our work and values, other information professionals may find it easier to attack the exercise on an incremental basis - taking the easy bits, or the bits where there are more committed staff first.

For us, as with other workers who choose to look critically at their performance, the disadvantages are that we can no longer hide our sins from each other or our users so easily. If you have an explicit statement saying that you must perform in a particular way, you must do so or know why you do not. This means that objectives must be formulated realistically and that staff must be prepared to work in this kind of limelight. However, it is our experience and that of quality assurance professionals, that many staff find it helpful to know why they are doing things, how well they are performing in relation to the norm, and how that contributes to the overall pattern of work. On the other hand, an explicit system of values allows library and information services to highlight areas where there is exceptional performance for their users and to find ways to bring resources or performance up to scratch in areas of poor service.

A practical disadvantage which we found following an extended period of unsettled staffing was that the objectives and performance measures must be set at realistic levels which allow sufficient flexibility to cope with some of the more obvious crises. When setting standards in a period of stability it can be tempting to disregard the effects of fluctuations in unit performance that can be caused by temporary variations in staffing or other aspects of the local situation.

Where next?

At the end of the exercise we felt that we had come up with an embryonic quality assurance system, which could be built up, over time, into a sophisticated managerial and performance tool. However, it is crucial to regard it as a dynamic system, in which the circumstances under which the service operates may change quite rapidly, and one which should be striving for continuous improvement in service to users. This has certainly proved to be true for the QAIS during the past year as 1990 has seen the introduction of fee-based services — initially in our enquiry service. We now have access to a number of software developments which make our computer-based work with the parent database more efficient, and the Quality Assurance Programme has specialist staff working in the areas of accreditation and consumer feedback whose information needs have to be supported. This means we have made some gains in working time, but these have not been sufficient to offset the extra information input and support required by our specialists. Also, fee-based services must be realistically priced, which means that we have to be looking to develop an increasingly accurate range of measures that allow us to determine what basic elements of the service cost, and what proportion of these might be recovered from our users. We must also look at cost recovery within the broader context of the King's Fund Centre philosophy on charging.

Conclusions

Making explicit our value base and service objectives has had a major impact on how we think about the QAIS. It has served to highlight areas where we need to do better or to focus the service in a different direction, but more often than not it showed us we were doing better than we thought, and that our performance measures were quite reasonable. It seems likely that our experience, although we are a national service operating in a narrowly defined subject area, would be similar to that of other small but more broadly-based library and information services. To date, setting objectives, standards and performance guidelines has been a relatively simple process and writing about our experiences in this way has made them seem more complex than they seemed at the time. We hope readers will forgive us for making the process sound complex. We have tried to highlight some of the arguments which other small libraries and information services might wish

to consider. We hope that our experience will encourage other information
workers to have a go.

Acknowledgements

Grateful acknowledgements are given to Tessa Brooks, Director of the Quality Assurance Programme and to Christopher Cuninghame and Guy Robin-
son, both former Assistant Information Officers, in the development of the
objectives and for their input to this paper.

Notes

[1] DHSS-DATA is the computerised database of the libraries of the Departments of Health and Social Security. It was established in 1983, and covers a
wide range of material relating to the management of health and social services and social security. It is available through a commercial database host
DATA-STAR [at 5th Floor, The Plaza Suite, 114 Jermyn Street, London
SW1Y 6HJ] who can offer more information about their complete service.

[2] *QUALITY ASSURANCE ABSTRACTS* are produced jointly by the
QAIS and the Department of Health Library. The bulletin is published
bi-monthly by the Department of Health, costing £14.00 p.a. in 1990. An
order form is available from the QAIS, Kings Fund Centre for Health Services
Development, 126 Albert Street, London NW1 7NF, or subscriptions may
be placed [cash with order] with the Department of Health Subscriptions
Unit [DPSU] at P.O. Box 21, Stanmore, HA7 1AY

[3] QAIS ENQUIRY SERVICE - customised reading lists and other information are provided on request on all aspects of quality assurance and
"quality" issues in health care. A fee [maximum of £15.00] per subject
search is charged and more information about the service can be obtained
from the Information Officer [QAIS] at the King's Fund Centre.